5/96 - Historical

EXTENSILE EXPOSURE

First Edition . . . *August* 1945
Reprinted . . . . *April* 1946
Reprinted . . . . *January* 1948

EXTENSILE
EXPOSURE

applied to

LIMB SURGERY

by

ARNOLD K. HENRY

M.B., Dubl.; M.Ch.(Hon.), Cairo; F.R.C.S.I.

Emeritus Professor of Clinical Surgery in the
University of Egypt; Professor of Anatomy
in the Royal College of Surgeons, Ireland

" 'tis not so deep as a well, nor so wide as a church door;
but . . . 'twill serve."

FIRST EDITION
(SECOND REPRINT)

BALTIMORE
THE WILLIAMS AND WILKINS COMPANY
1948

To
the Memory
of
R. S. Dobbin

αἰεὶ γάρ τε φέρει μειλίγματα θυμοῦ.

Made and Printed in Great Britain.

CONTENTS

PREFACE

EXPOSURE that will vie effectively with the " great arsenal of chance " must be a match for every shift, and therefore have a range, *extensile*, like the tongue of the chameleon to reach where it requires. This book, accordingly, seeks to enlarge the scope of certain set and parcelled methods of approach. It deals with means in which my confidence has grown from using them myself and watching others try them. And while a smooth success with first attempts pleased all concerned, mistakes (made as they were by persons of intelligence) proved real auxiliaries : they marked exactly what was ill-conceived or insufficiently described, and gave the chance for second thoughts—a chance these pages strive to seize.

Bone carries our anatomy and forms its central fact, and bone wherever possible is made the core of each exposure. Even the few confined to nerves and vessels bring in a glimpse of skeleton ; and some of these (though well rehearsed in other books and easily accessible) are borrowed here again. They form the roots from which exposures spread, and serve—like roots—to bind irrelative surroundings. The presence, too, of things so instantly attractive has let me note where charm may breed a moth-and-lamp effect that makes us " strut to our confusion."

The page who sings in *As You Like It* is correct : " hawking, or spitting, or saying we are hoarse " are only prologues to a bad voice ; and books, like songs, should be their own interpreters. But it is rare that one unaided person can write, print, illustrate and publish them. So debts alone may justify a preface ; and mine are large. My secretary, Mrs A. Wenham Brown—as quietly concerned for " a mistake in the dust of a butterfly's wing as in the disk of the sun "—has given deft, invaluable help at every stage, and latterly with indexing. Miss Zita Stead, the artist, adds to her gift the knowledge gained from actual dissection— a rare concurrence, used by her with scrupulous regard. Then, too, I have been fortunate to meet with a collaborator at once so expert, sterling and considerate as Mr Charles Macmillan, of Messrs E. & S. Livingstone Ltd., my publishers ; he puts a Scottish heart into his work.

To Professor J. H. Dible and the staff of his department I venture to express my gratitude for opportunities of contact with a welcome, stimulating climate—the evidence and birthright of a university. Dr J. Pritchard, too, at the Department of Anatomy, St. Mary's Hospital, has given me much friendly help.

That excellent technician, Mr J. Robson (now in the R.A.F.), has earned my special thanks, together with his friend, Mr V. Willmott, a very skilled photographer : their cheerful courtesy, and that of Section Commander C. Ward, was aid indeed.

The text in a superlative degree owes weeding and correction to my wife.

Lastly, a debt is due throughout to surgeons from every quarter of the Commonwealth. In friendly groups they formed (unwittingly) a panel whose jurors brought me verdicts ; and so these pages print what seemed to win, if not their full, unqualified approval, at least an *imprimatur*. Should I be wrong in that belief, the process of acquiring illusion for once sits smiling to the memory.

ARNOLD K. HENRY.

July, 1945.

INTRODUCTION

NOMENCLATURE

. . . d'abord la clarté, puis encore la clarté et enfin la clarté.
                                                    —ANATOLE FRANCE.

*Throughout the world in general—and, notably, in that of those who think and
write—I find it only in the ratio of the diamond to the mass of the planet.*
                                                    —PAUL VALÉRY.

A NEW nomenclature has recently appeared amongst
anatomists—the third in thirty years; and so, for men
of different age, a class to-day in operative surgery is
something like a class in Babel: one does not speak to it
collectively.[1]

I hold no brief for any terminology; the new, the old, the
Basle have each their points. The new, for instance, turns from
the vague " axillary " nerve of Basle back to the old and graphic
circumflex. But change which darkens what was clear is less
commendable. The trunk, for instance, that we knew (and still
know well) as musculospiral, ended by forking into branches
named respectively the " radial " and " posterior interosseous.".
This trunk then fell in line with continental usage and became
the radial of Basle nomenclature; its terminal divisions, too,
were well described as " deep " and " superficial." The third
and new nomenclature confounds the trunk and superficial
branch, and *both* are now called " radial." With that peculiar
precedent of lost distinction the internal popliteal nerve (*alias*
the tibial, *alias* the medial popliteal) might easily—in mounds
of new editions—be called " sciatic."

An opportunity is ripening; like us, America and the
Dominions have now had time to sift the question of nomenclature in English. Is it too much to hope that any joint,
definitive agreement will bear convincing signatures which prove

---

[1] This flux is not peculiar to anatomy. Dons have it too; Hilaire Belloc records the fact:
" They have turned the pronunciation of Latin (whereof we might have made a common
tongue for general intercourse) quite upside down, consonants and vowels and diphthongs,
so that my contemporaries can remember at least three quite different ways of pronouncing
the simplest Latin phrase, three different fashions in the short space of a human life.
Perhaps a fourth is coming." For Dons, he adds, are capable of anything.

it acceptable to those who work in *live* anatomy ? Till then let criticisms rain, but may there be a truce to efforts at establishing parochial adjustments !

And meanwhile with Herodotus, who cared for clarity and was (like us) unsettled by kaleidoscopic terms, " I shall continue to employ the names which custom sanctions,"—names which I know our surgeons understand. So without fear of puzzling anyone I say " the upper end " of humerus, or, if I wish, its " proximal extremity." Nor shall I waive the right to use " inner " and " outer " ; " internal to," " external to " ; " inwards " or " outwards." " Medial " and " lateral " are useful words ; I shall employ them too, but not *ad nauseam* ; the English tongue resents a curb, and answers best when reined discreetly. Perhaps for reasons similar the French (who then had much to lose) refused to bow the knee to ' Basle.'

We recognise[1] at once the inner aspect of the thigh (or arm or leg), so why not speak of it ? And though the present fiat of anatomists restricts the term of " inner surface " to linings of the hollow organs, yet, if I write that certain nerves lie to the inner side of arteries, will someone really think they lie within the lumen ?

Such things, of course, are trifles weighed against the fact that every terminology has pockets of resistance to surgical approach. And these (within the boundary of my text) I am resolved to liquidate.

ON CERTAIN AIDS DERIVED FROM STRUCTURAL ARRANGEMENT

The operations of our intellect tend to geometry.
—HENRI BERGSON.

Que ferions nous sans le secours de ce qui n'existe pas ? . . . Les mythes sont les âmes de nos actions.—PAUL VALÉRY.

Some general considerations.—Few that invade the structure of anatomy are artists ; the great majority take care, for the convenience of their memories, to force its details into shapes of Euclid—triangles, quadrilaterals, circles of peculiar form. The few (and they are very few) need no such framework ; like painters who from scribbled notes of " green " or " yellow " produce a replica with tone and shade in exquisite gradation,

---

[1] *Recognise, recognize* ; *mobilise, mobilize*, etc. The *Oxford English Dictionary* is strong for " z." But Pater who was ' Oxford ' allows the " s "—like Quiller-Couch of Oxford *and* of Cambridge. I shall abide by *Kent's* uncompromising verdict (*King Lear*, Act II, Sc. 2).

these few as easily recall the un-Euclidean visage of anatomy and deal with it as though by instinct.

The many (like myself) who fail to share the artist's gift are glad of aids—despised by those who do not need them. And here the targets for their scorn are plentiful : these pages nowhere scruple to include whatever crutch or simile or dodge has proved its worth repeatedly to groups or individuals. I am, indeed, convinced (like Tristram Shandy's father) that there exists " a North-west passage to the intellectual world, and that the soul of man has shorter ways of going to work, in furnishing itself with knowledge and instruction." Things, therefore, such as satellites, loop-holes, half-sleeves, shoulder-straps, cloaks, seams, leashes, bucket-handles, lids, sandwiches, V's and manual mnemonics—these myths are rife throughout. Let us examine one or two more closely.

The half-sleeve.—By this I do not mean a sleeve cut short across but one divided lengthwise, covering subjacent structures somewhat in the way a cradle covers patients suffering from shock. We come upon such half-sleeve muscular investments behind the shaft of humerus ; in front of the femur ; at the back of the calf. In each half-sleeve there is a seam to find and rip —giving the latter word precise, housewifely meaning, remote from crime or even butchery.

Loop-holes.—A muscle in the space between attachments must have a portion of its belly ' free,' that is to say continuous with everything surrounding it in such a way as to allow of normal action and harmless instrumental separation. These parts when short and when we separate them out will form the boundary of a loop-hole which may give initial access to a deep and perilous position. A useful fingerbreadth of biceps, for example, close to the distal end of femur, lies free behind the intermuscular septum ; a touch will make the belly bound a loop-hole which can then be widened safely.

Satellites.—This term of satellite denotes a state of linked companionship, like that of median nerve with the sublimis belly, or of its ulnar neighbour with profundus ; for, coming from behind into the forearm, the latter trunk is fastened to the deeper muscle. A satellite relation thus implies reciprocal divorce from other structures. Specific application of this knowledge— of union as distinct from mere proximity—prevents much futile groping (pp. 59, 123).

Other aids.—We should contrive to wring the utmost benefit

from details of anatomy ; examples of this kind of exploitation
are scattered through the text. Contributors in this respect
are planes of cleavage, and I try to show how best to find them.
Other aids abound. A bursa, for example, may help to make our
surgical approach as smooth and easy as the gliding of its own

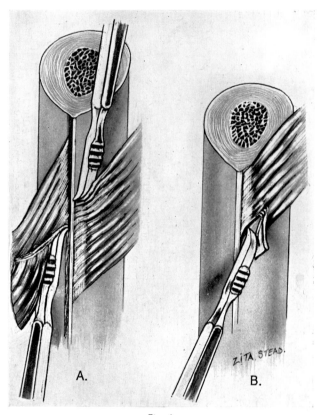

Fig. 1

The stripping angle

Work the rugine into the acute angle which fibres of muscle or
interosseous membrane make with bone. (B shows how the
rugine tears into a muscle when used in the reverse direction
—against the obtuse angle.)

tendon (p. 60). Or fibres from another source may cross and
bind the grain, say of the popliteus—a muscle that when split
gives only meagre access. The crossing fibres then will mark
a line for sectioning the muscle and also stop the creep of sutures
through the grain (p. 144). A structure tethered on a single
border will move more readily towards its tether, uncovering
objectives deep to it ; so to reach them easily, divide the skin

along the border *opposite* the tether (p. 148). Angles of attachment help or impede the separation of fibres from bone. And muscles grasped and moved across their fixed companions provide the surgeon with a kind of tangible mnemonic which helps him for incising skin and separating structures (*The Lancet*, 1940, **1**, 125). Allusion to these angles and mobilities are frequent in the text and need some further explanation.

THE ACUTE OR STRIPPING ANGLE.—A shaft is stripped most easily of fibres, whether of muscle or of interosseous membrane, by working the edge of the rugine into the *acute* angle which the fibres make with bone at their attachment. Used in the opposite direction—towards the obtuse angle—the rugine tends to leave the bone and tear into muscle or membrane (Fig. 1). There is a two-way application of this principle when we expose the shaft of femur ; here the stripping angle opens proximally for adductors, distally for vasti. Then, too, on the fibula the muscles have a stripping angle opposite to that of interosseous membrane (p. 163).

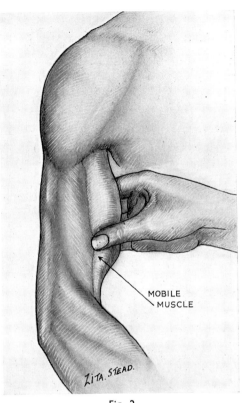

MOBILE
MUSCLE

Fig. 2
Comparative muscle mobility
The biceps—fixed at either end—can easily be moved across the widely fastened breadth of brachialis. Thus, for exposure of the front of humerus, the *fingers* can discover (in spite of fat or swelling) exactly where we should incise and where to find the part of brachialis that separates shaft from skin.

COMPARATIVE MUSCLE MOBILITY.[1]—We can make use before and during operation of the facility of moving certain muscles across their much more fixed companions. Lines of incision may thus be ascertained where fat, posture or swelling might cause disorientation ; and planes of cleavage, too, can be located by this means. Before we cut down on the front of the humeral

[1] *The Lancet*, 1940, **1**, 125.

shaft we first shall grasp and move the free biceps belly across the widely fixed attachment of brachialis fibres, and thus find out exactly where to split the portion of this latter muscle which separates the skin from bone (Fig. 2). Behind the humerus we move the long free head of triceps in relation to the lateral fixed head, and so find out exactly where to split the loose half-sleeve with which this pair of superficial elements covers the musculo-spiral nerve and deeper head (p. 17). A wad of three long bellies flanks the radius and must be mobilised before we clear its shaft. The fingers move these muscles to and fro *en masse* across the supinator and against the fixed extensor bellies. So we can feel out lines for skin incision and planes of cleavage, front and back : in front, when we approach the shaft of radius (p. 61) ; behind, in looking for the posterior interosseous nerve—the deep (terminal) branch of radial in Basle nomenclature (p. 74). The stiff edge, too, of lateral intermuscular septum (a structure vital to one femoral exposure) is recognised by moving the lax mass of biceps across its greater fixity (p. 121). Lastly, for access to ulnar bursa, mid-palmar space or deep terminal branch of ulnar nerve, finger and thumb locate and move abductor digiti quinti in the free margin of the hypothenar mass.

Separation of closely related structures.—We shall in general contrive to separate these structures cleanly if we begin their separation at the place where they begin to separate—a precept which Fiolle and Delmas stress throughout a book that is the breath of present-day exposure.[1] This principle has widespread application : it works, I find, as smoothly in the chest as in the limbs. The flimsy sacs of pleura tear unless we start divorcing them where they divorce themselves to clothe the apex of the lungs (*see* " A Technique for Removing Pulmonary Emboli," *The Lancet*, 1940, **1**, 349). So on the limbs we look for places of divergence : a member of a bundle turns aside, or crowded bellies fan towards their tendons.

Sometimes, as we shall see, a pair of thumbs (well gloved, of course,) laid lengthwise on a pair of bellies will open up a twisting plane of separation—technique that will be blamed by those who have not learnt to trust the hand, the quintessential root— in every sense—of surgery.

[1] J. Fiolle and J. Delmas, *Surgical Exposure of the Deep-seated Blood Vessels*, London, 1921.

THE CUTTING OF CUTANEOUS NERVES

So when the buckled girder
Lets down the grinding span,
The blame for loss, or murder,
Is laid upon the man.
Not on the Stuff—the Man !

—RUDYARD KIPLING.

Incisions must divide the *branches* of cutaneous nerves, but they should aim to cut as few as possible and should at least avoid the major stems. Once in a while painful neuroma follows their section or their injury, giving the patient little rest and sometimes ruining a life. These cases, though infrequent, are living accusations. We should endeavour not to swell their ranks.

Incisions will be planned accordingly. I have twice lately met with scars of operation on the knee, U-shaped and classical, giving rise to sharp and frequent pain, in one case lasting seven years—an extra reason for discarding crooked cuts. We can as easily excise the knee—or do whatever else we must—through an incision that is straight and *shorter* than the U. (A piece of string bent and unbent will illustrate the point.) Apart from nerves, however, the U that cuts the blood supply on either side of skin tends to produce a marginal necrosis.

In certain regions it will not be possible to heed these atraumatic counsels : a large exposure in the neck or shoulder *must* cut some large cutaneous nerves, rarely indeed with after-penalties, though I have seen two patients recently whose broken clavicles had injured branches from the neck, causing neuralgic pain. And often, in the fingers, trigger-spots arise from tiny twigs in necessary scars.

These then are counsels of perfection. Yet, if we look, we recognise abundant opportunities of sparing nerves, which those in daily contact with post-operative limbs will try to seize. Some, too, may find (as I believe) that these cutaneous disasters, though commoner in people with a certain temperament, can yet assail the balanced individual. To *all* of these unfortunates the pain is real, and little satisfaction can be got by blaming them for faults of therapy or chance.

Such lesions should be treated urgently before the pain takes root within the thalamus, thence to wear slowly out ; or else wear out the patient. For when the thalamus is sick no surgery can cure—except the guillotine.

Sometimes in early cases we succeed immediately. A procaine infiltration of the trigger-spot, if followed up at once by movement, may stop the pain; and even (rarely) after long duration. (This happened with the painful knee I mentioned, which was cured for months by two injections—till the patient fell and bruised the scar.) But failure, too, is common. Sometimes resection works a charm (it cured my two clavicular neuralgics) —or sympathectomy. They often fail. There is no rule whatever. Therefore (once more!) let us respect cutaneous nerves.

TECHNIQUE

I shall guard my asepsis as a girl should guard her virginity.
—A colleague, thirty years ago.

This modest note may find a welcome now that bones and joints will come the way of general surgeons—stirring perhaps unquiet memories; taboo and half-forgotten ritual; no-touch technique for knees, long instruments for femurs. But though the need for care is paramount, there *is* need also for simplicity. The common sense of Moynihan has left us safe and easy methods which retain the service of our best auxiliary, the hand, and let its well-gloved fingers touch both joint and bone. A twenty-year experience of these measures in general surgery and in major orthopædics has made me certain that a single ritual works well in either field.

The skin as enemy.—Moynihan would not permit the outer surface of a glove to touch the skin at all—either the hands of surgeons or the skin of patients: he branded contact as a fault, however well the hands were cleaned or skin prepared. And while for many years we all have learnt to don our gloves, touching their inner surface only, the gain is often lost by using them to handle patients' skin. If we avoid this fault throughout the operation, a sterile and undamaged glove remains as sterile as a metal tool, and may, I know, " explore a knee joint . . . with impunity " (Moynihan, *British Journal of Surgery*, 1920, **8**, 29).

But gloves (as L. G. Gunn once said of cats when sutures broke) " ain't what they used to be "; so it may now be wise to smear, in case of accident, some dettol cream upon the hands

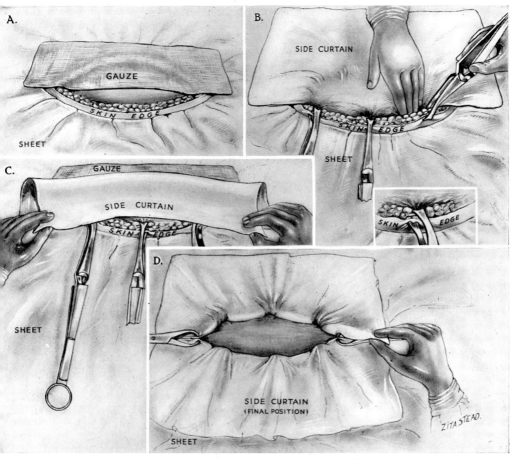

Fig. 3

Application of a side curtain. (A sterile sheet is already in place)

A. Screen the patch of bare skin at one side of the wound with a piece of gauze.

B. Lay the curtain flat on the gauze and bring the edge of the curtain to the *opposite* edge of the wound. Depress the edge of the curtain deep to the whole edge of the wound before applying clips. (That is vital ; otherwise skin will bulge between them.) Fix this depressed edge of curtain with clips so that one jaw of each clip fastens the cloth to subcutaneous tissue while the other bites directly on to the surface of the skin (see inset).

C. Lift the free opposite edge of curtain, and cover the clips by turning the curtain over through two right angles. Discard the gauze, treating it as soiled, *having touched skin.* (The second curtain, applied in the same way, is screened from skin by the first and needs no gauze.)

D. The two curtains in position. Terminal clips can be hidden at will, as shown on the right side.

before the gloves go on.[1]   Or should the skin resent it, as does mine, wear *two* pair, using cream upon the first.

(This attitude to skin implies that we discard each knife used for dividing it—with other tools that touch—and then take fresh ones to continue.)

Masks.—The parts of these that screen the nose and mouth should be impermeable. The best are made entirely of cellophane (except for fittings on the face and ears) ; but pockets stitched to common gauze varieties of mask will hold thin sheets of cellophane and screen effectively.

Marking the skin for final closure, though not concerned directly with asepsis, allows of perfect apposition. The scratches of a fine *round*-bodied needle should cross proposed incisions ; a cutting needle is apt to leave a scar. These slight marks will help in closing any operation wound ; they are essential when the parts take new position during closure, a lesson sharply driven home by suturing an unscratched case of old luxation of the shoulder.

Side or wound curtains.—The use of these is almost universal, though they are often so applied that wads of naked skin bulge into view between the towel-clips. Fig. 3 and its legend show a technique due to my former colleagues, Richard Slattery and Faïd Yusry, and I shall only touch here on the value of Michel clips for fastening these curtains. *Clips have no handles*, a special virtue when one has to curtain neighbouring incisions, say on the foot. (Some recent makes, I find, have lost their grip, reverting to the flaccid types of thirty years ago that came unstuck when patients moved.)

LONG INCISIONS

For neurovascular bundles.—The use of wide approach for dealing thoroughly with nerves and vessels needs no defence, but tends to slip at times into oblivion. These neurovascular

---

[1] A friend whose skin was harbouring staphylococci has told me that use of dettol cream allowed him to complete his operating sessions with hands and *wrists* both negative to culture tests. In this connection, too, the observation made by L. A. Weed and Jessie L. Groves at Indiana University Medical Centre is relevant. One or more gloves were found perforated at the close of almost three-quarters of the operations performed— viz. after 3409 operations out of a total 4549 (*Surgery, Gynecology and Obstetrics*, 1942, **75**, 661). There is, however, still on many sides an unashamed solicitation of infection : the septic case (apart from all emergency) is often touched, or even dressed, with naked hands by persons who will presently affect aseptic ritual—a sight that stirs the gorge of those conditioned otherwise.

bundles are moored extensively along the limb by frequent offsets ; they are impossible to mobilise through short incisions, nor can they be explored. ' Closed ' lesions of the vessels as a rule in swollen, freshly injured limbs demand a long incision ; for often they are multiple and may occur in great variety, though signs are few and point to nothing certain but the need for intervention. Then, too, a neurovascular bundle—like that behind the knee—can bar the way to an objective and must be widely mobilised before we can retract it safely.

For bones.—The long incision is essential in exposing bones. I do not know of any principle of surgery less easy to instil ; yet on its proper application depends success with compound fractures that reach us *early*—the rule to-day aside from stress of battle. In these fresh accidents a septic outcome has, I have found, been variously viewed by those concerned. To some it was a normal happening ; to some a case of surgical misfortune ; to some again it seemed the sign of slipshod treatment for which they felt a plain and personal responsibility. Of late the rediscovery of Pirogoff's great finding—so useful in its proper place—that septic limbs can stink their way to health in plaster, has innocently been the source of a defeatist question : What harm if early fractures suppurate ? The answer is : The curse of sepsis when it grips a bone ; or (on another plane of evil), the waste of time—and beds.

We can frustrate this curse, almost with certainty, by thorough early cleansing, in company with secondary measures ; so that an open fracture which has skin to cover it should normally be " simple " in a week, while those devoid of skin are rescued from the drag of suppuration. Incisions, therefore, must be long enough for us to find and clear away both dirt and damaged tissue.

If we have reason to suspect that dirt has reached the bone, then we must scrutinise the site of fracture—especially the central portion of the broken ends. For this too-frequently neglected step cut a three-quarters of the length of shaft will only just suffice, even with bones so near the surface as the tibia ; and thus, if dirt engrains the ends, it can be lightly chiselled off. But if we do not look, it is impossible to *know* these broken ends have not been soiled ; and if we leave them soiled (whether from negligence or grim extraneous necessity) we sabotage the operation. Bone, in the suspect case, will thus decide the length of our incisions : those long enough to let us bring the ends for scrutiny are long enough to let us cleanse the wound throughout.

A NOTE ON EARLY OPEN FRACTURE.—The background of a damaging remark made to me lately by a surgeon, young, travelled, well-informed and capable, evoked these most unfashionable paragraphs. " Our generation," he said, " associates the treatment of compound fracture with a bad smell." This turned my thoughts again to Egypt where certain ancient Greeks, too faithfully disguised as seals, once lay in ambush and suffered terribly till rescued from the deadly stench.

These fractures were among the commonest emergencies of Cairo. Their treatment in my unit was carried out by colleagues who, since 1926, believed themselves at fault if they fell short of turning well over 90 per cent. of open lesions into clean or simple fractures. This work, I feel, deserves a record. For it seems clear to me that if some sixteen years ago such high success could be achieved with soiled, subtropic fractures in patients, often underfed or sapped by parasites, to-day with newer means and better nourishment the incidence of sepsis in early open fractures should be negligible—a thing I failed to note since leaving Egypt.

Our method in the Cairo unit was based on pages of Lejars'—remembered from a 1903 edition. It was enhanced by what I learnt in 1917-18 from Richard Stoney's notable results with bipp, dilute and harmless—another very grateful recollection.

We did not use a plaster case till 1931 for open fractures, but only splints or gutters, yet our success, considered in the light of absent sepsis and rapid union, was just as excellent without as with : it is the cleansing, not the plaster, that decides.

The cleansing of the wound and of the bone are dealt with in the text ; here I shall merely stress the fact that any slackness in preparing normal skin was always paid for by an upward trend of sepsis : our best results were got when wound and skin alike were cleaned with equal thoroughness. We learnt to treat the limb *en masse*—as if for sterile operation on a joint— and, using ether first, we painted all the skin with brilliant green—a 1 per cent. solution in 30 per cent. alcohol.

The need for mild antiseptics in the wound.—No matter how well we execute the task of cleansing a wound—not forgetting the routine but economic resection of its original damaged border—our cleansing is only macroscopic, and many dirty points remain unseen. It is, I believe, for this microscopic residue that mild antiseptics have their use in recent compound fracture. Those that served best in my time with the unit (1925-36) were : (1) the dilute non-toxic bipp of Stoney's formula—well rubbed in after sousing the cleansed wound with ether ; (2) a 1 per cent. aqueous solution of mercurochrome freely applied—combined, as we shall see, with bipp.

On not quite closing the wound.—In 1927—just when we felt most confident—I learnt from a septicæmic death in a long, completely successful series, never again to close the full length of these wounds ; and in our lines of suture we thenceforth left an opening opposite the site of fracture. Through this inch-wide gap a wick of sterile gauze or bandage impregnated with dilute bipp reached from bone to skin. If loss of deeper tissues left dead space, we used the wick to fill the cavity. This packing of the cavity with a loose bulk of heavily bipped wick, inimical to growth of organisms, is merely an example of the old and far too much forgotten Mikulicz device for drainage ; it leaves no breeding pools nor burrows for discharge to loiter in, but makes instead—all round the well-bipped pack—a film, unstagnant and unstinking, that flows directly to the surface.

We then covered the line of suture with an equally well-bipped pad, and the limb was put in plaster, leaving a long window opposite the pad. After forty-eight hours we withdrew the wick and renewed the pad. (For the preparation of dilute bipp see the footnote, p. 142.)

Denuded fractures.—A wide destruction of the tissues is found in certain compound fractures and leaves exposed a length of bare and broken bone. The cleansing of such wounds when dirt-ingrained, by the slow process of picking up and cutting off each bit of damaged tissue takes more time than some of these patients can well stand.

The task compares in difficulty with piecemeal cleansing at low tide of rocks spread with seaweed ; when the tide flows, wide mats will rise on *pedicles* and lend themselves to clearance. Water from a tap at any place with clean supplies will serve to simulate the tide : under the stream the damaged tissues float on stalks, and these are then snipped off, in rapid contrast with the weary plucking of a sheet of scum.

The *force*, too, of the stream will help to clean the wound ; its whole might is brought to bear on every part in turn by narrowing the outflow from tap or tube. This simple method —far from original but little used—was put in hand for me by Faïd Yusry in 1931.

Success began, I think, to smile on us one day in 1925 when I decided with my friend Handusa to rank the compound fractures with acute abdominal emergencies. That put their treatment in the able hands of five successive colleagues—Ahmed Handusa first, then Edward Sadek, Faïd Yusry, Lotfy Abdelsamie, Mohammed el Zeneini. When I see better results than theirs in open fractures on as large a scale with any other method I shall wish to try it.

For muscles.—We need a long incision, too, for mobilising certain muscles—the wad of bellies, notably, that screen the lateral face of radius. This wad takes origin above the elbow ; the knife must therefore follow it and reach well up the *arm* to let us view the radius widely in the forearm.

OPENING DEEP FASCIA

Division of the fascial envelope needs something of the care we spend on dura mater ; for otherwise we plough the muscles, wreck planes of cleavage, and even wound a shallow-lying popliteal nerve or radial vessel—in swollen limbs especially.

One useful method is to grasp the fascia with forceps and make a cut to introduce the tip of Mayo scissors. The tip keeps close against the fascia and opens slightly on the flat ; it then alternately, in little steps, advances and divides. If it goes far enough to rip the envelope " in one," the contents, too, are ripped.

MEASUREMENTS

Those damned dots.—LORD RANDOLPH CHURCHILL.

Throughout this book a use is made of fingerbreadths and handbreadths [1] ; sometimes of spans, which may be generous or otherwise. They have advantages : the means of making them are always with us, and those I shall describe have stood the test of years. Their own variety appears to chime with the vagaries of anatomy that mock our text-book decimals—a consonance I always find amazing ; for students, surgeons, patients and cadavers vary remarkably in size and shape.

---

[1] The hyphens are left out ; they may be dropped in compound words (says Fowler) as soon as the novelty of the combination has worn off. And here this argument applies : Hippocrates employed the fingerbreadth, and this, no doubt, he " went an' took—the same as us."

EXPOSURES IN THE UPPER LIMB

. . . et ayme plus souvent a les saisir par quelque lustre inusité.—MONTAIGNE.

OUR first attack accords with the caprice of wounds. Choosing the arm we " pinch it to the bone " by an unwonted aspect and thus obtain the windfall of a type exposure.

This comes conveniently and well equipped to illustrate the Introduction. We find at once the means for wide inclusive access : a muscle we can move and steer by ; a V, a half-sleeve and seam, a bucket-handle ; useful mobilities and friendly dispositions. But terminology has seen to it that these auxiliaries (like persons in the fairy-tale) are neutralised and checked from full cooperation. They are, in fact, bewitched.

APPROACH TO THE WHOLE BACK OF THE HUMERAL SHAFT EXPOSING FROM BEHIND THE NEUROVASCULAR BUNDLES OF THE ARM

His opinion, in this matter, was, That there was a strange kind of magick bias, which good or bad names, as he called them, irresistibly impressed.
—TRISTRAM SHANDY.

The three heads of triceps.—A blight of terminology conceals the simple plan of triceps, a plan which is the key to this approach. And so we have the queer, ingrained confusion of a long head (unquestionably long but medial too) companioned by a head called " medial " or " inner " which has—in man at least—no title to the name. For the main bulk of so-called " medial head " springs, not as one might think, from medial parts of humerus, but (as Albinus notes)[1] from the whole breadth : and, what is more, the head lies covered by its fellows. A curious example of nomenclature—amusing, if its " magick bias " were not a drag impressed on intervention.

When once we break that spell, the plan of triceps shows in full simplicity : two heads—the long which leaves the scapula, the lateral which springs from humerus—are *superficial*. And these

14

heads joining V-wise form a loose half-sleeve that shrouds the third (Fig. 4). This third head, therefore,—miscalled the " inner " or " medial "—is certainly the *deep* head of triceps.[1]

Viewed in this way the whole muscle becomes a kind of wish-fulfilment : the very details of anatomy are on our side.

[1] Since that was written I found my view already held by a professional anatomist who long ago had called the head *deep*. Use of the term *medial head* " is apt," he wrote, " to give rise to some misconception of its nature and position " (T. H. Bryce (1923), in Quain's *Elements of Anatomy*, London, 11th edition, vol. iv, Part II, p. 124). No echo followed this gentle understatement ; but in a recent issue of the *Sunday Times* I came (with some surprise) on the appropriate remark : " If Dons," it quoted, " are not even accurate, what the hell are they ? "

Albinus saw the facts quite clearly ; the magnificent folio of *Tabulæ* from Dobbin's great collection shows the deep head displayed by the cutting away of its two companions " quibus subjacet " ; and the note on Fig. 7, tab. XIX (1747) adds : " Et initio suo occupat amplitudinem ossis." Albinus calls the deep head *brachialis externus*, the counterpart for him of our plain brachialis—a muscle which he qualifies *internus*. (This seems confusing till you let your arm hang naturally down ; then you will see the force of his description.) So, for Albinus the triceps has two layers : (1) a superficial, bicipital layer whose long head is our long head and whose short head is our lateral ; (2) a deep layer.

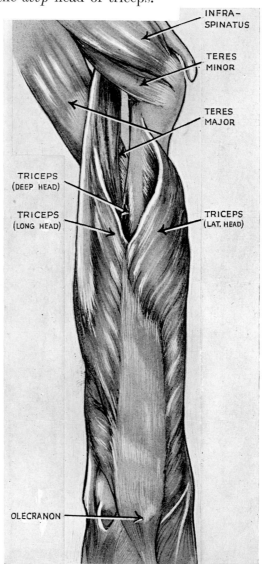

Fig. 4

The three heads of triceps

The superficial heads (the long and lateral) meet in a V ; they spread and form a loose half-sleeve almost completely hiding the third and *deep* head of triceps (called perversely ' medial ' or ' inner ').
The deltoid has been removed. Note how it would slope across and cover the proximal part of the lateral head.

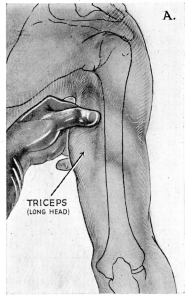

A.

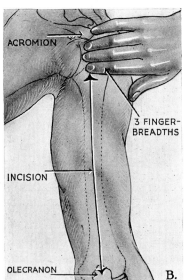

B.

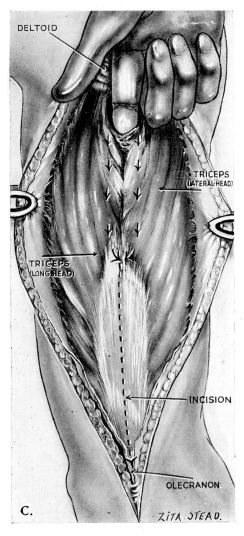

DELTOID

TRICEPS
(LATERAL HEAD)

TRICEPS
(LONG HEAD)

INCISION

OLECRANON

C.

ZITA STEAD.

ACROMION

3 FINGER-
BREADTHS

INCISION

OLECRANON

TRICEPS
(LONG HEAD)

Fig. 5

A. **Finding the long head of triceps.**—This is your guide (1) for incising the skin ; (2) for finding the V-shaped opening of the half-sleeve. Grasp it where it goes from scapula to arm and move it on its stationary neighbours (deltoid and lateral head). Divide the skin and fascia close beside its outer edge ; the entrance to the sleeve lies *there*. (If you lose touch with longus you tend to lose your way between deltoid and lateral head.)

B. The **skin incision** begins beside the outer edge of the long head three fingerbreadths distal to the acromion. It goes down to olecranon.

C. **Opening the seam of the half-sleeve.**—Keep the finger close to the outer side of the long head and enter the V. Ease the loose sleeve off underlying structures. Begin the separation of long and lateral heads gently with the finger ; continue with the knife, dividing the oblique fibres of lateral head at their attachment to the tendinous lamina which is developed—as Albinus notes—by longus in the depth of triceps. This lamina looks forwards and out (see Fig. 6).

16

THE OPERATION

Finding the long head.—With the patient face-down we abduct the arm and look first for the long head of triceps, our guide in this approach.[1] Luckily the long head is far more mobile than the neighbouring deltoid and lateral head, and we need merely grasp and move it in order to distinguish it from either (Fig. 5, A).

Incision.—This follows the outer edge of the long head beginning three fingerbreadths below the acromial angle and going straight down to the olecranon (Fig. 5, B). When the skin has been divided, we shall again grasp and move the *proximal* part of the long head, so that we may open the deep fascia close to its outer side. Here the finger will enter the V-shaped meeting-place of long and lateral heads, and working down in contact

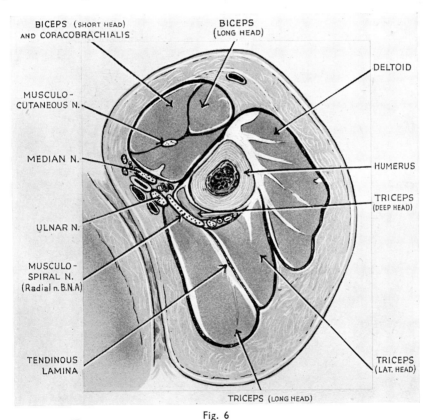

Fig. 6
The tendinous lamina developed by the long head
It marks the seam of the half-sleeve. Note, too, how the ulnar nerve lies at the sharp, anterior edge of the long head. This guiding edge is separated from the nerve by thin fascia.

---

[1] The V-shaped junction of the long and lateral heads may show as a depression on a thin subject with the arm abducted in the face-down posture.

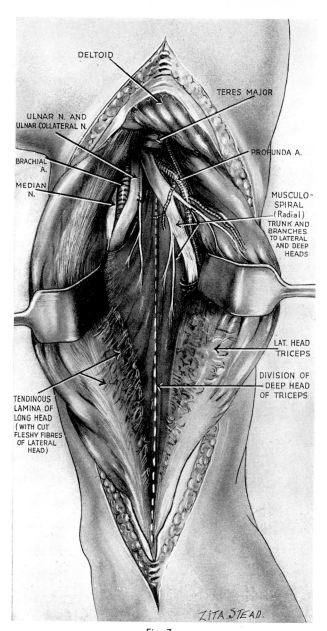

DELTOID

TERES MAJOR

ULNAR N. AND
ULNAR COLLATERAL N.

PROFUNDA A.

BRACHIAL A.

MEDIAN N.

MUSCULO-
SPIRAL
(Radial)
TRUNK AND
BRANCHES
TO LATERAL
AND DEEP
HEADS

LAT. HEAD
TRICEPS

DIVISION OF
DEEP HEAD
OF TRICEPS

TENDINOUS
LAMINA OF
LONG HEAD
(WITH CUT
FLESHY FIBRES
OF LATERAL
HEAD)

ZITA STEAD.

Fig. 7

The half-sleeve opened

The seam is ' ripped ' ; the two halves of the sleeve (the superficial heads—long and lateral) are separated, exposing the slanting
neurovascular bundle. This consists of musculospiral nerve and
profunda vessels ; it crosses the deep head, which clothes the
humerus behind much as brachialis clothes it in front. Some four
fingerbreadths of the main neurovascular bundle (ulnar and median
nerves, brachial vessels) show in the space between long head and
deep. Note the useful gap between the two parallel musculospiral
twigs, leaving room to split the deep head. (The medial twig is
the ulnar collateral.) Note and take care of the branch to the
lateral head of triceps.

18

with the long head will presently hook into the loose half-sleeve
(Fig. 5, c). But we must be sure to keep in contact with the
guiding belly ; the finger otherwise may open the wrong plane
and lose its way between lateral head and overlying deltoid.
That is the first pitfall.

Separation of the superficial heads (the long and lateral).—
A finger hooked into the V-shaped opening lifts the sleeve from
what lies under, and then begins to rip the seam that marks the
meeting of these heads. But
soon we need a knife (Fig.
5, c), for fleshy fibres of the
lateral head slope down to
join a shining lamina which
the long head develops in
the depth of triceps (Figs. 6
and 7).[1]

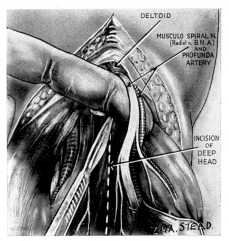

Fig. 8

Raise the oblique bundle like a bucket-handle,
working from below, and lift it clear of the deep
head. The deep head can then be split lengthwise from end to end. (The branch to lateral
head must be picked up with the main bundle ;
it is likely to be cut if the bundle is mobilised
from the proximal edge.)

The bright face of this
oblique ' intrinsic ' tendon is
the plane for clean separation.

Opening the half-sleeve we
find the large bundle consisting of musculospiral nerve
(the radial of B.N.A.) and
profunda vessels, a slanting
band thinly divorced from
bone by the deep head of
triceps (Fig. 7). And if we
raise the bundle gently like
a bucket - handle and loop
it back (Fig. 8), we then can pass the knife beneath, split
the deep head lengthwise and reach almost the whole shaft
from behind (Fig. 9, A).

Mobilising the musculospiral bundle.—Begin at the distal
edge of the bundle on the medial side of the wound and work
outwards. The lateral head of triceps receives a large nerve which
runs a more transverse course than its parent trunk, and so is
widely separate from the slanting bundle (Fig. 7). We must not

---

[1] This detail was familiar to Albinus : " It is impossible to show in this figure "—6 of tab.
XIX—" how the long head develops (*efficiat*) a wide tendon on the side next (*a parte*)
the lateral head, and how fibres of the lateral head reach it—just as on the *surface* of
triceps (*extrinsecus*) fibres of the long head reach the lateral." (I have used our term
" the lateral " for the head Albinus calls " the short.")

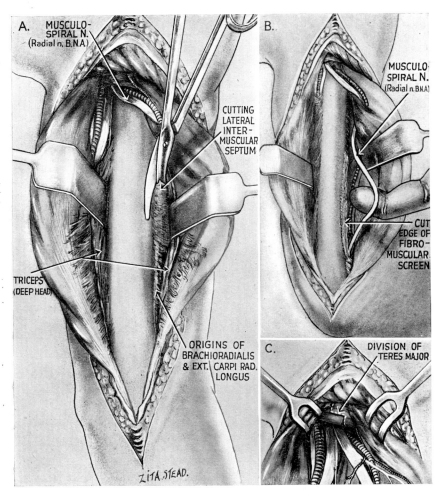

Fig. 9

A. The humeral shaft exposed from behind.—The two halves of the deep head have been peeled off the bone and retracted.

B. Extending the back view of the musculospiral (or radial) nerve.—(The outer half of the deep head must first be fully raised from the back and outer edge of the shaft. This brings the small tongue of muscle which parts musculospiral from bone (Fig. 6) across behind the nerve.) *Distally*, divide the fibromuscular screen that hides the nerve. This screen consists of the lateral septum together with the flat origins of brachioradialis and extensor carpi radialis longus which are *in front* of it. Note that the distal part of the septum is drawn *as if transparent*, to show these origins.

C. *Proximally*, divide the flat band of teres major plus latissimus tendon. (Note the Z-shaped cut for sound repair.) Adduct the arm to relax the musculospiral which can then be drawn out like a loop (as in B).

fail to loop the branch and bundle up together (Fig. 8), for if we overlook the branch, it will most probably be cut—a frequent fault in making this exposure. (An ascending leash from profunda vessels may cross the field obliquely and go deep to deltoid (Figs. 7 and 10); sometimes it is large.)

Splitting the deep head.—Even the nerves to this part of triceps befriend our purpose : the inner half of the deep head is supplied by the fine ulnar collateral, a musculospiral (radial) twig that is often closely bound to the ulnar trunk and was long mistaken for a true ulnar branch (Fig. 7); the outer half has a stronger parallel twig (which also innervates the anconeus). Thus we can split the deep head between two longitudinal branches (Figs. 7 and 8). But the knife should keep close to the more lateral of these and aim for the olecranon; otherwise we may injure the ulnar nerve which sometimes bends outwards before reaching the elbow.[1]

The posterior approach to the humeral shaft resembles that for exposing the anterior, homologous face of the femur. There, too, a loose half-sleeve of muscle covers a deep head crossed by a neurovascular bundle; there, too, we rip a seam, loop the bundle and split the deep head to reach bone.

EXTENDING THE POSTERIOR VIEW OF THE MUSCULOSPIRAL (OR RADIAL) NERVE.[2]—When the outer half of the deep head is fully raised from the back of the humerus the lateral intermuscular septum comes into view and—in company with the flat thin origins of brachioradialis and extensor carpi radialis longus— screens off the musculospiral nerve which goes in front. Divide this fibromuscular screen as close as possible to bone and so avoid the twigs to muscle (Fig. 9, A); then relax the nerve by adducting the arm (Fig. 9, B). That will let us deal with three more inches of musculospiral trunk, a surplus gain which often saves the nuisance of making fresh incision to find and liberate the nerve in front.

At the proximal part of the wound a similar length of musculospiral can be won by dividing the compound band of

---

[1] *This curve is dangerous.* I have seen the ulnar trunk divided during the exposure ; but fortunately, so far, in the dead.

[2] " Musculospiral " appears again as an alternative. The recent imposition of " radial " on stem and branch alike has robbed the word of meaning for those long since acclimatised to both the previous terminologies. And some (who weathered each) would willingly agree with Pater that since " all progress of the mind consists for the most part in differentiation . . . it is surely the stupidest of losses to confuse things which right reason has put asunder, to lose the sense of achieved distinctions."

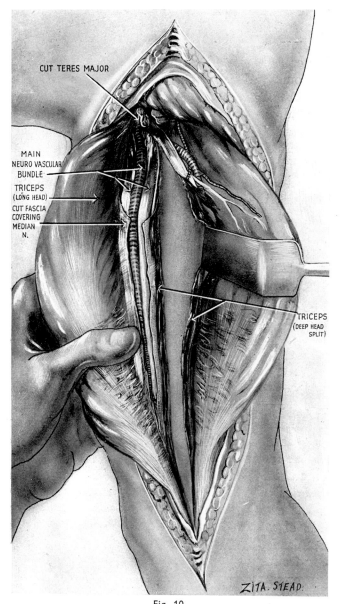

Fig. 10

**The posterior exposure of humerus extended to
the main neurovascular bundle of the arm**

Separate the long head from the deep, and thus enlarge the upper
space through which the bundle is already visible ; a screen of fascia
must also be divided. Grasp the arm as in the figure (but through
towels). Work the bundle up into the wound, using your finger-tips
to bring it round the inner side of the deep head. (The median nerve
sometimes sticks to the front of the brachial artery.) Access is easy
and room sufficient to explore the bundle and recognise its frequent
abnormalities (high division of the artery, etc.).

latissimus and teres major tendons, after easing the ulnar and musculospiral nerves safely away from its anterior face. A Z-shaped section of this band (Fig. 9, c)—made tense by abducting the arm—will favour strong repair.

THE MAIN NEUROVASCULAR BUNDLE OF THE ARM SEEN FROM THE BACK.—The brachial vessels and median nerve are easily explored in this posterior approach, for when we separate the long head of triceps fully from the lateral, some 4 in. of main bundle are seen in the upper part of the field (Fig. 7). But farther down the arm the bundle is first veiled by a sheet of fascia and afterwards concealed by the deep head of triceps, in front of which it rests. Turn then to this deep head and separate the long head from it right down the arm. Through the covering towels grasp and gently squeeze the inner side of the arm in such a way that the tips of the fingers will bring the bundle round the inner side of the deep head and up into the wound. Thus we can deal from behind with the great anterior nerves and vessels (Fig. 10).

APPROACH TO THE FRONT OF HUMERUS
WITH EXTENSIONS TO ITS JOINTS
TO THE FOREARM AXILLA AND ROOT OF NECK

During a surgical exposure important neurovascular structures are spared in one of two ways: either we seek them out for protection, or else avoid them completely. So, in our access to the back of humerus we find the musculospiral nerve and loop it clear, whereas with *frontal* intervention on the shaft, the nerve will—if we wish—remain concealed and undisturbed. And this exposure of the front of humerus provides, as we shall see, a base for exploration of the parts at either end— the joints, axilla, neck, and forearm.

ANATOMY

The *proximal* part of the bone is concealed in front by deltoid fibres coming from the lesser curve of clavicle (Fig. 11); the

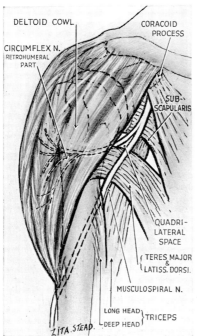

Fig. 11

The deltoid cowl whose front must be
swung back for wide access to the top
of shaft and to the shoulder joint.
(*Lateral* incisions that split the deltoid
threaten the circumflex nerve.)

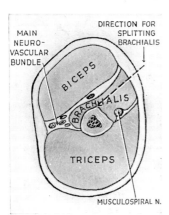

Fig. 13

Cross-section through mid-third
of arm, showing the outer flank
of brachialis which is bare of
biceps. This flank is split in the
direction of the pointer to expose
the distal half of humerus in front.
The cut slopes in to reach the
middle line of shaft. The musculospiral is safe.

muscle forms a thick unyielding
cowl which gives when pulled
aside a grudging revelation of bone
and shoulder joint ; and that will
often be the last successful thing
it does. So, for a *wide* approach
we mobilise the cowl in front and
turn it harmlessly away.

Clothing the *distal* reach of shaft
are longitudinal fibres of brachialis
belly whose outer flank, left free of
biceps, comes to the surface in

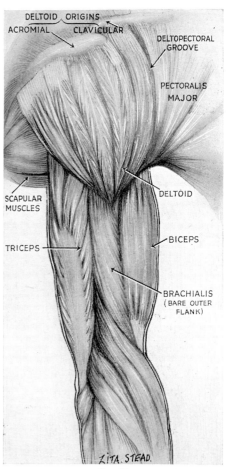

Fig. 12

The wide, bare *outer* flank of brachialis alone
separates skin from shaft in the distal half
of the arm (see also Fig. 13).

surprising width (Fig. 12). Here, then,—on the outer side of the arm—a single muscle (with its fascial coat) separates skin from bone ; and here we shall attack the shaft through this uncovered flank of brachialis (Fig. 13).

The musculospiral (or radial) nerve.—The solid V of deltoid insertion fits down into a hollow V of brachialis, behind whose rearward limb lies the musculospiral nerve (Fig. 14) ; thus, we detach the limb (or separate its fibres) to find the nerve infallibly—a fingerbreadth below the deltoid eminence. But that is as we wish : the nerve need not be seen at all.

The *cutaneous trunk of musculocutaneous* curves forward at the outer edge of biceps just where the belly joins the tendon of insertion (Fig. 15). One of the outer cutaneous filaments is likely to be cut in the upper third of the forearm, though care will leave it running like a thread across the wound. (Main musculocutaneous branches to muscle are high up under cover of the inner part of biceps belly.)

The *cephalic vein* which follows the outer border of biceps and the inner border of deltoid enters the deep fascia in the lower third of the arm. It receives two or more lateral tributaries which must be divided. A humeral branch of the thoracoacromial artery accompanies the vein in the deltopectoral groove, and gives twigs to both muscles ; the knife, therefore, cutting down on bone, should keep clear of this vascular gutter (Fig. 15) and go instead through fibres of the deltoid that form its outer lip.

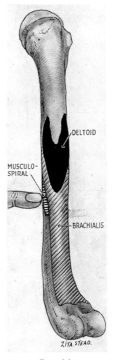

Fig. 14

Anterolateral view of the humerus showing how the solid V of deltoid insertion fits into the hollow V of brachialis. The musculospiral (radial) nerve lies behind the outer limb of brachialis V and can be found a fingerbreadth below the apex of the deltoid eminence (see also Fig. 23).

From these facts it appears that our incision to expose the front of humerus will skirt the outer side of the cephalic vein—below, where it follows the outer edge of biceps ; above, in the deltopectoral groove ; so we shall keep the knife a modest fingerbreadth *lateral* to the course we map for the vessel (Fig. 15). In the distal reach, however, no mere line will always guide the surgeon ; fat or swelling may affect disorientation, and I have made (and often seen) the slip of

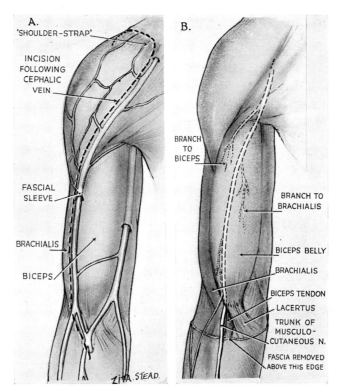

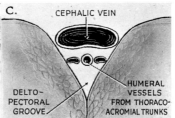

Fig. 15

A. The cephalic vein skirts the outer edge of biceps and the inner edge of deltoid. Incisions to expose the front of humerus follow the vein along its outer side. The broken line *above* the delto-pectoral groove maps out the arching part, or 'shoulder-strap.'

B. Note how the chief cutaneous trunk of musculocutaneous appears where biceps belly joins with biceps tendon.

C. Cross-section showing that the deltopectoral groove is a vascular gutter. We shall avoid it and cut lengthwise through its deltoid lip to reach the bone.

cutting through the biceps belly in mistake for brachialis flank. We therefore grasp the front of the lax anæsthetised arm (Fig. 16) and move the free biceps belly across the fixed mass of brachialis. *Then* we can locate the outer edge of biceps and with it the cephalic.

We shall see, in a moment, how to find and follow the course of the deltopectoral groove in exposing the proximal part of humerus.

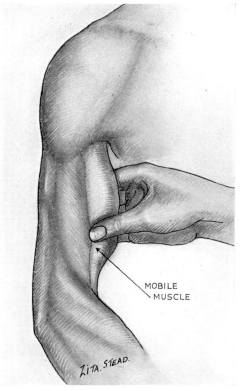

Fig. 16

Find the edge of biceps by moving its mobile belly across the fixed mass of brachialis. With this guide we can (1) place our skin incision for the distal part of the shaft a fingerbreadth from biceps ; (2) avoid the cephalic vein ; and (3) find the flank of brachialis, which (with its fascial coats) alone separates skin from shaft. This flank we shall split, directing the cut to the *midline* of humerus (see Fig. 13).

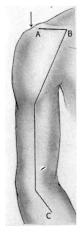

Fig. 17

The incision originally described for humeral exposure. The crooked proximal part (designed to give room to mobilise the clavicular origin of deltoid) is now replaced by a 'shoulder-strap' (see Fig. 18). The figure is retained to show the useful 'step-down' at the arrow which marks the acromioclavicular joint.

THE PROXIMAL PART OF HUMERUS AND THE SHOULDER JOINT

The incision I once used for this exposure was acutely angled at the outer third of the clavicle in order to give plenty of room : first, for mobilising the deltoid cowl and turning it out of the way ; then, at the close of intervention, to allow easy fastening of the cowl back into place (Fig. 17).[1] But crooked cuts in skin have three

[1] *British Journal of Surgery*, 1924, **12**, 84.

faults : they are troublesome to fit with side-curtains ; they
are troublesome to close, and thirdly, they compromise healing.
For many years, therefore, I have used incisions that cross the
shoulder archwise from front to back (see *Irish Journal of Medical
Science*, 1927, p. 634).

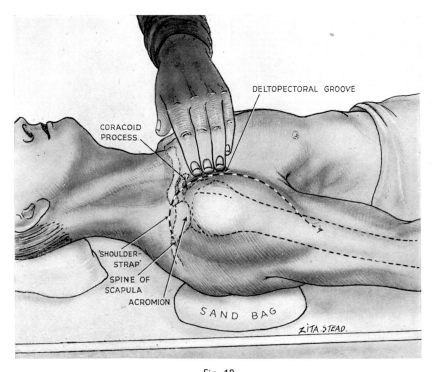

Fig. 18

**Position and shoulder-strap incision for exposing the proximal
part of humerus**

Make the *back* of the shoulder accessible to the knife by putting a flat sandbag 5 in. square
by 2 in. thick under the lower part of scapula on the side of operation. The bag must
not obscure the scapular spine. Note how the coracoid tip is thrust into prominence.
The knife goes through skin only, from deltoid eminence to scapular spine ; it follows
the direction of deltopectoral groove and crosses the coracoid top before arching over
the shoulder. *To find the deltopectoral groove* the hand lies flat on the chest and slides
out over the lax front of pectoralis major. The tips of the fingers strike the firm, oblique
edge of deltoid ; the groove lies under them.

Position.—Care is required to make the *back* of the shoulder
accessible to the knife. The patient lies with a flat sand-bag,
5 in. square by 2 in. thick, under the *lower* part of the scapula
on the side of operation. The bag lifts the shoulder sufficiently
to show the scapular spine, and also thrusts the tip of the
coracoid process forward into helpful prominence (Fig. 18).

The shoulder-strap incision.[1]—
If we confine exposure either to
the joint or the proximal part of
humerus, the 'shoulder-strap'
descends no farther than the distal
end of deltoid ; so we shall first
locate the deltopectoral groove,
whose course the knife will follow.
Sliding the fingers out towards the
limb across the hollow face of pectoralis we touch a firm obliquity of
deltoid edge (Fig. 18). The groove
is there, beneath the finger-tips.
The knife—which cuts no deeper
than subcutaneous fat—will follow
up the groove to reach the tip of
coracoid ; then it will cut straight
on over the shoulder down to the
level of the spine of scapula—or,
of course, in reverse, according to
the side of the limb, or manual
convenience (Fig. 18).

Open the deep fascia along the
whole length of groove close to
its outer edge and look for the
cephalic vein which occupies its
channel. The knife can then avoid
the groove (with all the vessels
it contains) and split instead its
deltoid margin lengthwise from end

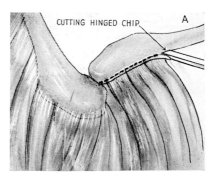

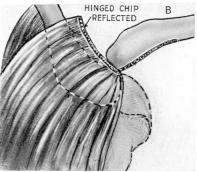

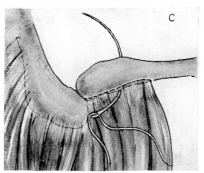

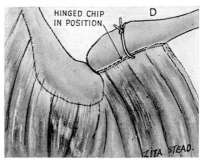

Fig. 19

Mobilising the front of deltoid

After reflecting skin, turn the deltoid out
on a hinged chip cut from the lesser curve
of clavicle, A and B. The deltoid origin
can be reconstructed with a single
ligature passed on a large curved needle,
C, and tied, D. Note how the chisel—
seated on its *bevel* to prevent undue
penetration—cuts out as far as the
acromioclavicular joint, marked by a
'step-down' (see Fig. 17).

[1] I had ventured without hesitation to call this a shoulder-strap incision till I realised the
adjective came from a word used sometimes of bands running from tip to collar *along*
the shoulder. Let the term stand ; my intention is plain to a majority : no woman will
question it.

to end.   This useful detail—due to G. A. Mason (*British Journal of Surgery*, 1929, **17**, 30)—divides a negligible strand of muscle from its nerve.   A small reflection of the shoulder skin gives access to the piece of deltoid that springs from the outer third of clavicle.

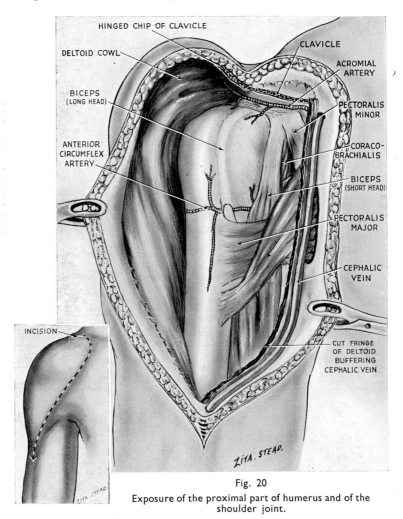

Fig. 20
Exposure of the proximal part of humerus and of the shoulder joint.

Mobilising the front of the deltoid.—Divide the fascia and periosteum on the upper face of this outer third near the front of the bone.   Then detach a mere shaving of the edge that carries the deltoid origin.   If you are right-handed stand ' below ' the level of the patient's shoulder on his right side ; ' above ' it on his left.[1] Use a chisel and cut out as far as the acromioclavicular joint

[1] Or,—if you prefer,—let your stance in respect of the right shoulder be caudad : of the left, cephalad.

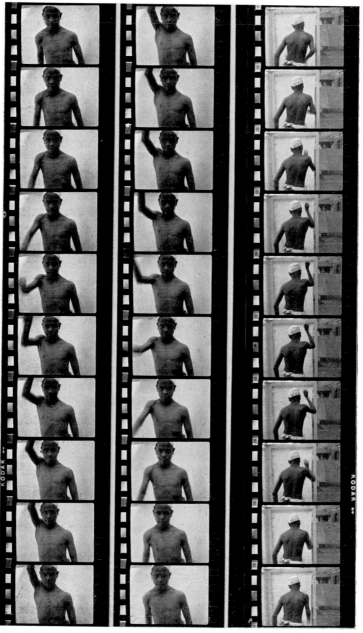

Fig. 21

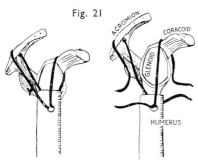

ACROMION
CORACOID
GLENOID
HUMERUS

To show the function of a limb after the deltoid has been mobilised and reconstituted. In this case the proximal fifth of humerus was resected for tumour, and the shaft slung with fascial strips to the scapula (see inset). Ten years later the function remained excellent. The left and middle columns are consecutive pictures from a film; the patient, who worked in brass, raises his right arm, keeps it raised, and then lowers it. The right-hand column shows a complete hammering movement.

(Figs. 19 and 20). It is very easy to cut deep into clavicle and so remove too much bone. Seat the tool therefore on its *bevel*, and use it—like the blade of a carpenter's plane—to separate the edge only (Fig. 19).

The front part of the deltoid cowl can now be turned out on a hinged piece of clavicle, like a curtain on a rod. But the wide prospect we gain in this way is disappointing at first sight if we forget the spread of bursa that remains to mask (and be removed from) our objectives (Fig. 20).

After dealing with bone or joint a single suture passed through the muscle and round the clavicle with a large curved needle will lash the small piece of bone back into place and so reconstitute the deltoid origin (Fig. 19).[1] (The bony chip which carries deltoid need by no means be unbroken ; I have often cut instead a band of mere contiguous flakes ; and these united quickly with the clavicle, leaving the deltoid function quite intact.)

THE DISTAL PART OF THE HUMERUS (BELOW THE DELTOID LEVEL)

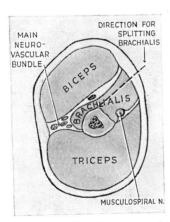

Fig. 22

Cross-section through mid-third of arm, showing the outer flank of brachialis which is bare of biceps. This flank is split in the direction of the pointer to expose the distal half of humerus in front. The cut slopes in to reach the *middle line* of shaft. The musculo-spiral is safe.

Guiding our incision by testing for comparative mobility (Fig. 16), we keep the knife a slender fingerbreadth lateral to the edge of biceps, and so respect the vein ; then we continue four fingerbreadths into the upper third of the forearm, curving a little in towards the middle line. Here we must open deep fascia with extra care, especially in swollen forearms. The swelling seems to thrust the radial vessels (which are, I notice, often slit in normal limbs) still further into danger. Surgeons, too, will take a pride in rescuing the lateral cutaneous twig of musculocutaneous which runs in surface fat (Fig. 15). A longitudinal cut is then directed through the bare outer flank of brachialis, which we identify again by moving biceps

---

[1] I still describe this way of mobilising and reconstituting the deltoid origin, which served me well through twenty years in dealing with the following conditions : old subcoracoid luxations ; osteoclastoma of the humeral head treated by resecting the proximal fifth

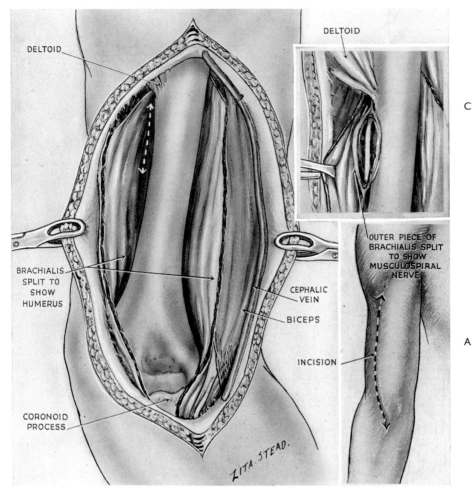

Fig. 23

Distal exposure of the humerus

A. The skin incision. B. When we have split brachialis as in Fig. 22, a partial flexion of the elbow transforms the split into a wide and shallow wound. If exploration of the elbow joint is not required, check the cut two fingerbreadths above the epicondyles. Musculospiral meanwhile is safe and out of sight. Should you wish to find the nerve, a touch with Mayo scissors parts the screen of brachialis one fingerbreadth below the deltoid eminence (B and C).

---

of the humerus and suspending the rest with fascia to coracoid process and acromion (see Fig. 21, from the *Irish Journal of Medical Science*, Oct. 1927, reproduced here through the courtesy of my friend the Editor, Mr. W. D. Doolin); recent subglenoid luxations of the shoulder with fractures comminuting the proximal parts of humerus. In every case exposure was completely satisfactory; in none did the chip fail to unite with clavicle, and none has required removal of wire, thread or catgut.

I have often wondered, however, if a subperiosteal detachment of deltoid would be compatible with the sound function I got after cutting the chip. And recently I had the fortune to hear from Lt.-Col. H. A. Brittain, R.A.M.C., that excellent results will follow. More sutures must be used to tie the muscle back in place than when it swings out on a rod; but that is no objection.

3

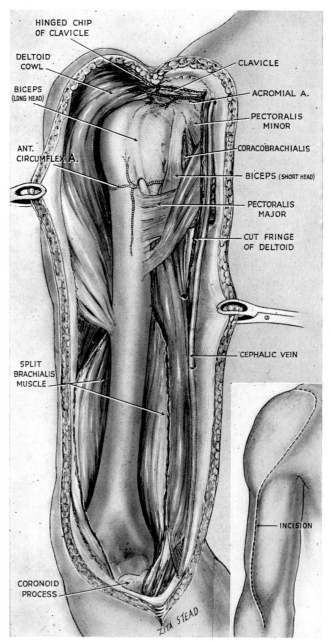

Fig. 24

Complete anterior exposure of the humerus, embracing shoulder and elbow joints, is obtained by combining the proximal and distal exposures in one procedure. The inset shows the full incision. Musculospiral does not appear unless we wish (see Fig. 23).

over it; the knife enters the flank a fingerbreadth lateral to the biceps edge and goes obliquely in to reach the front of the bone *at the middle line*—a vital emphasis (Fig. 22). (I have only once seen the nerve injured in scores of humeral exposures— then by a glancing, misdirected cut, wide of the ample target.) The outer strip of brachialis, thus separated, forms a buffer protecting the musculospiral (or radial) nerve from the rugine. The nerve is not seen if the front only of humeral shaft is exposed; the back, too, can be cleared safely while the nerve is concealed. But (should the surgeon wish) the musculospiral, in adults, is always found one fingerbreadth distal to the deltoid eminence by gentle blunt dissection through the buffering slip of brachialis (Fig. 23). Light pressure on this buffer removes the nerve sufficiently from contact with the shaft to give a rugine access. (This facultative finding of the nerve was plain in the original account (*loc. cit.*), but has been missed in later adaptations.)

The brachialis may be split to just within two fingerbreadths of the epicondyles without entering the elbow joint. Watch for sharp bleeding from a vein divided in the upper fibres. The bone, seen through the split, lies, in extension of the limb, deep and unworkable. Flexion of the elbow to a right angle transforms this appearance, relaxing the muscles and leaving the bone widely accessible in a shallow wound (Fig. 23).[1]

The elbow joint.—This joint can be opened—and even excised from in front—by a further splitting of brachialis. The tip of the coronoid process and the trochlea are at once visible; the capitulum and head of radius appear with adequate retraction.

After a distal approach, extension of the elbow before suturing the fascia will close of itself the wide wound in brachialis.

The whole front of humerus can be laid bare by combining the proximal and distal approach (Fig. 24); and we can, of course, expose any segment by using shorter lengths of the full-length incision. But these should not be short.

If, therefore, it is possible to reach objectives (sequestra are the commonest example) *without* hinging back the deltoid, we need not hinge it back,—a sentence one would like to think superfluous.

[1] For a continuation of distal exposure of humerus into antecubital fossa see p. 49.

EXPOSURE OF THE PROXIMAL PART OF HUMERUS COMBINED WITH AXILLO-CERVICAL EXTENSIONS TO NERVES AND VESSELS

Some fifteen years ago with Major D. Bowie, then surgical specialist to Cairo Command, I saw a case of fracture-dislocation of the shoulder showing complete brachial palsy. We had thus to explore the bone, the joint and proximal parts of all the brachial nerves. The shoulder-strap incision described above (Fig. 18), combined with detachment of a clavicular chip (Fig. 19), served well ; bone and joint were dealt with, and, after dividing the tendon of pectoralis major, each nerve was seen and fortunately found intact. The following account will give a sort of formula for multiple procedures of the kind.

AXILLARY EXTENSION OF THE PROXIMAL APPROACH TO HUMERUS.—The shoulder joint and upper part of humerus are first exposed (see p. 27). Then, when the deltoid is turned back, divide the tendon of pectoralis major close to its insertion and draw the muscle inwards (Fig. 25). The loose fascia now seen spreading between the divergent coracoid origins of pectoralis minor and coracobrachialis covers the main neurovascular bundle of the axilla. Open the fascia near the coracobrachial belly avoiding the musculocutaneous nerve which enters a medial *groove* on that muscle two fingerbreadths below the coracoid ; farther down, the nerve tunnels through the muscle belly.[1]

When we have opened the loose axillary fascia it is quite easy to take the wrong path—even after careful warning—and be lured by the inviting space between bone and the composite band formed by short head of biceps plus coracobrachialis (Fig. 25). Resist that lure and keep dissection *medial* to the band. The nerves lie there in easily remembered grouping round the vessels (Fig. 25).

Some special points deserve a reference. The *median nerve* can as a rule be found, even with eyes shut, by Farabeuf's simple expedient—drawing the pulp of a finger across the main axillary bundle towards coracobrachialis ; the nerve comes with the finger and leaves the artery bare (Fig. 25). The circumflex and musculo-

---

[1] Pictures in text-books of anatomy show the musculocutaneous dissected out of the coracobrachial groove ; they therefore stress a relation of nerve to muscle which begins only at the *tunnel*. That, I think, is why we learn to expect the musculocutaneous in a third-stage axillary ligation, and why we seldom find it : the nerve has sunk into the groove and left the median to skirt the lateral edge of neurovascular bundle.

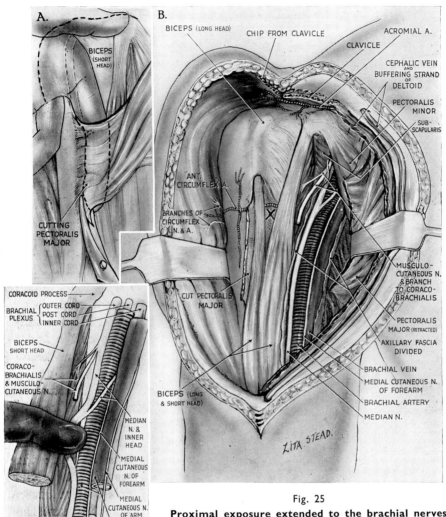

Fig. 25

Proximal exposure extended to the brachial nerves

A. The pectoralis major divided. B. The resulting exposure. X marks the pitfall to avoid when defining the neurovascular bundle—the tempting much-frequented interval between short head of biceps and humerus. (The bundle is, of course, *medial* to the common mass comprising biceps head and coracobrachialis.) C shows the relation of nerves to the double-barrelled lie of vein and artery in the axilla : the medial cutaneous nerve of forearm occupies the groove that demarcates the barrels in front ; the hinder groove conceals the ulnar nerve ; median overlies the outer border of the artery and is accompanied by musculo-cutaneous, while medial cutaneous of the *arm* is on the inner border of the vein. C also shows Farabeuf's ' blindfold ' method of locating the axillary part of median nerve.

spiral nerves spring from the hinder cord ; they thus lie deeper than the rest and come less easily to hand.

The circumflex nerve.—This nerve, considered for a surgical exposure, has here two parts—axillary and retrohumeral (Fig. 26).

The *axillary portion* which suffers most from injury lies deep ; and having failed on more than one occasion to find it quickly, I learnt at length to recognise it blindfold—defining in the first place with a finger the thick mass of main neurovascular bundle.

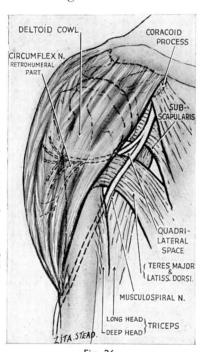

Fig. 26

The posterior cord forks into circumflex and musculospiral nerves. Each nerve has an axillary and a retrohumeral segment. The quadrilateral space is seen.

LOCATION OF THE AXILLARY PART OF CIRCUMFLEX BY TOUCH. —Stand behind the top of the patient's shoulder and use your right index for his left side, your left for his right. Place the tip of the finger on the tip of the coracoid ; aim into the angle formed by the divergence of pectoralis minor and coracobrachialis. Slide the finger obliquely—down, in and back—across the coracoid tip as far as the proximal interphalangeal joint. The tip of the finger penetrates soft areolar tissue above the level of the bundle, and, slanting down behind it, stops against the front of the subscapularis (Fig. 27). Now turn your index and hook the distal phalanx gently out towards the arm ; the thick strand thus caught by the pulp of the finger is the circumflex bundle : the nerve lies next the finger ; in front of the nerve are the posterior circumflex vessels.

But when we find this portion of the circumflex we have achieved a mere location : it lies as yet too deep, and seems too short, for useful intervention. Not till the clavicle is cut at the responsive point (p. 42), letting the limb fall outwards, will a workable length of nerve come near enough the surface for convenience.

The *retrohumeral part of the circumflex* disappears through the quadrilateral space above the thumbwide band of latissimus and teres major tendons (Fig. 26). A finger easily enters the distal part of this space and follows the transverse course of the bundle round behind the humerus; it lies in a loose zone of cleavage between deltoid and surgical neck.

EXPOSURE OF THE RETROHUMERAL PART OF CIRCUMFLEX.—This portion of the nerve is only seen by further mobilising deltoid—first distally as far as the insertion; then at the proximal attachment.

Separation of the acromial origin of deltoid.—Leaving a strand to buffer the cephalic vein (p. 29) the whole deltoid hood is mobilised without division of its fibres, first by detaching the hinged clavicular

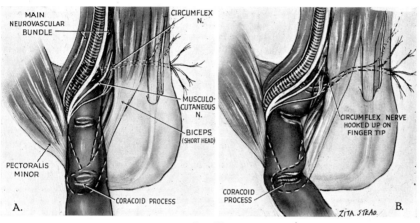

Fig. 27
Locating the axillary part of the circumflex nerve by touch

A. The index finger (the left for the right side—as in this figure—and *vice versa*) slides from above the patient's shoulder, on its palmar aspect, *across* the coracoid tip, *into* the angle between pectoralis minor and coracobrachialis, *behind* the main neurovascular bundle, viz. down, in and back. Stop the finger when its proximal interphalangeal joint covers the tip of coracoid. The distal phalanx has then reached subscapularis—the soft mass in front of scapula.

B. Now turn the finger out towards the arm. The distal phalanx hooks the nerve.

chip completely, and then by cutting off with a chisel the deltoid edge of acromion (Fig. 28). Adopt the stance employed for slicing off the deltoid chip (p. 30)—' below ' the patient's right shoulder; ' above ' his left. And once it bites into the bone, seat the chisel on its bevel (as in Fig. 19) and take the merest shaving from acromion, *except* at the acromial angle. Cut this angle off obliquely in such a way that when replaced it will fit firmly on the scapula. The whole bony margin—acromial plus clavicular—looks like a bent and sprawling U with one limb broken (Fig. 28, c). This separation is by no means difficult, but does demand most careful study of skeletal contour (Fig. 28) and gentle guidance of a *sharp* chisel. The

very wide exposure thus obtained (Fig. 29) should also find a use in
the rare case where mere *clavicular* detachment gives insufficient
access to the shoulder, and where as well we have the chance of
saving deltoid function.

The final restoration is extremely simple, for to secure it we
need only tie back into place the chip first cut from clavicle. A
single ligature will thus reconstitute the origin of deltoid—in front,
behind and at the side.

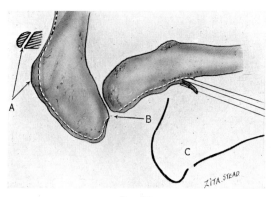

Fig. 28
**Separation of the deltoid origin extended to
acromion**

A. The acromial angle ; the broken line marks the
direction of the cut seen from above. The sagittal
section shows in diagram the *slope* of the cut which lets
the separated angle fit back later like a cap. B. The
' difficult ' corner between the bones—where it is
easy to drive the chisel *through* acromion instead of
round its edge. C. The outline of the cut seen from
above—a sprawling U with one limb broken. (The chips
from clavicle and acromion are linked across the joint by
ligament so that a single suture round the clavicle re-
constitutes the deltoid origin.)

The musculospiral nerve.—The musculospiral runs obliquely in
front of a useful landmark, the composite teres-latissimus tendon
which crosses the field four fingerbreadths below the coracoid tip.
The nerve lies, remember, like the circumflex, *behind* the main-
neurovascular bundle, shut off from it and bound by thin transparent fascia, so that when we draw the bundle inwards the
musculospiral is often left unmoved and visible (Fig. 30).

The vascular tether.—But first we may have to sever a short
leash of vessels that ties the bundle to the coracobrachial belly,
near the latissimus tendon. A finger travelling down the belly
catches the leash which comes either from brachial or profunda
vessels ; and since the leash is short these last are easily hooked

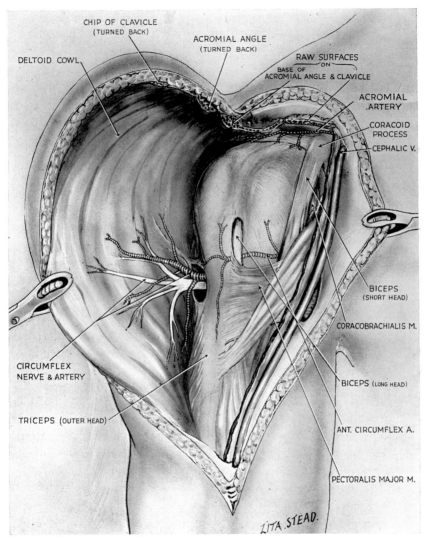

Fig. 29

Subtotal detachment of deltoid

Exposure of the retrohumeral part of circumflex obtained by detachment of the clavicular *plus* the acromial origins of deltoid. The wide, incidental, view of shoulder joint—front, side, and back—suggests further use for this subtotal deltoid separation. *One* ligature (placed as in Fig. 19, C) restores and clamps both origins.

up with it (Fig. 30). We shall do well, therefore, to separate and view the structures caught by the finger before dividing the leash, sparing of course the large profunda.

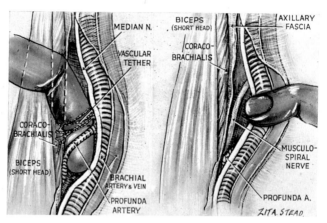

Fig. 30

A vascular tether binding the main bundle to coracobrachialis may need division before the bundle can be drawn aside to expose the musculospiral nerve. A finger hooked down the medial face of coracobrachialis picks up the tether—and sometimes the large profunda vessels with it. So look before you cut, and spare profunda.

THE CORDS OF BRACHIAL PLEXUS.—The cords from which the nerves arise are thoroughly exposed if the narrow, coracoid end of pectoralis minor is cut across.

EXTENDING THE EXPOSURE FROM THE AXILLA TO THE NECK.—For this the clavicle must be divided. The site made use of by Fiolle and Delmas affords a real seat of election, three fingerbreadths lateral to the sternal end (Fig. 31, Part 1). Division of the bone too far in threatens the subclavian vein which lies so dangerously close to the medial inch of clavicle; on the other hand, a section too far out leaves an inner piece of shaft whose overlap conceals our main objectives. The 'seat of election' corresponds in general to the outermost edge of the sternomastoid origin—a place to remember; for there the external jugular vein penetrates deep fascia; there, on a deeper level, we shall find the outer edge of scalenus anterior underlying that of sternomastoid—the two as if about to coincide in Euclid's mind.

When the clavicle is sectioned we can use the weight of the limb to lever the outer fragment from in front of the plexus.

Position and incision.—The field is opened by turning the patient's head and neck away, and pulling on the hand to bring his

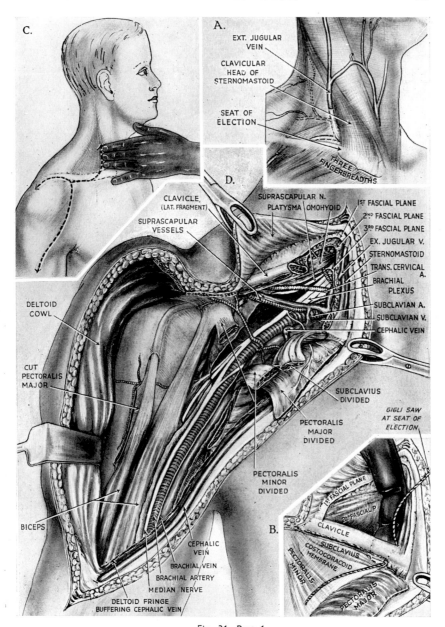

Fig. 31, Part 1

Exposure of nerves and vessels continued from axilla into neck by cutting through the clavicle

A and B. Seat of election for dividing clavicle, three fingerbreadths from the sternal end. It borders generally on the outer edge of sternomastoid—an edge which is displaced directly back would 'coincide' with that of scalenus. Note the relation of external jugular.

C. Incision for *unforeseen* extension from joint and axilla to neck, going in from the 'strap' to a fingerbreadth beyond the 'seat', and then up sternomastoid—a useful makeshift (*cf.* Fig. 31, Part 2).

D. The view after (1) dividing pectoralis major close to clavicle; (2) dividing pectoralis minor; (3) dividing clavicle itself; (4) drawing the limb clear of the table so that its *weight* will swing aside the outer fragment. This last manœuvre levers up the final tether (belly of subclavius). Cut through it, taking care to guard the sometimes formidable suprascapulars.

shoulder down. Then comes the question of incision. Supposing, for example, we have used a ' shoulder-strap ' and bared the joint, only to find that we must *add* an exploration of the root of neck, the requisite incision goes inward from the ' strap '—a second-best though workable procedure (Fig. 31, Part 1). But if we

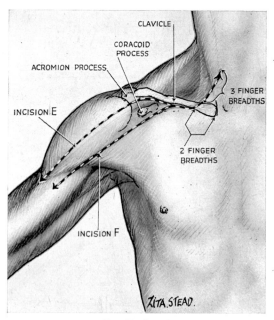

Fig. 31, Part 2

Skin incision for planned axillo-cervical approach

E. *For exposing axilla plus shoulder joint plus root of neck,* abduct the arm to straighten your cut. Divide skin length-wise over deltoid, aiming a thumbwidth *lateral* to the tip of coracoid. Curve the cut in along the lower edge of clavicle, and up, two fingerbreadths from sternum.
F. *For simple axillo-cervical approach* again abduct the arm. By-pass the joint with an incision curved like E, but aimed a thumbwidth *medial* to coracoid.
Incision E affords inclusive access to the joint (Fig. 19). Incision E or F leaves room for opening the pectoralis lid to the axilla ; then for dividing moorings of the clavicle—a barrier which, cut across, not only swings aside but lets the shoulder girdle turn and offer up the contents of axilla on the scapula, as on a plate.

plan combined exposure—whether of shoulder joint and neck with axilla, or merely of axilla with neck—then we shall make a single cut, placing it farther in or out, to let us by-pass or include the joint (Fig. 31, Part 2). Reflect skin sufficiently to show three things : the site for dividing clavicle ; the origin of pectoralis major lateral to that site ; the lower fourth of sternomastoid. Add—to expose the shoulder joint—the outer third of clavicle.

Division of pectoralis major and clavicle.—After severing the muscle near its humeral attachment we must divide it from the clavicle as far inwards as the place for bone section, so that presently the lateral fragment (which blocks our view of nerves and vessels) lies ready to be swung aside.

We now turn to the neck and open the most superficial of the three layers of deep cervical fascia close to this ' seat of election.' A finger introduced from above completes the isolation of the clavicle at the right spot. The instrument of choice for dividing the bone is a Gigli saw.[1]

Then, if we bring the limb well over the edge of the table, its weight will lever up the outer piece of clavicle and stretch the belly of subclavius. This we must divide without dividing vessels —variously termed the transverse scapular [2] or suprascapular— whose long *retroclavicular* course (stressed by the Baron Boyer in Napoleon's time) runs close behind subclavius. Many to-day, I notice, find their site and magnitude surprising. But John Bell, who lived his anatomy, often saw the artery (which frequently springs from the third stage of subclavian) " large, very long, tortuous like the splenic artery, and almost equalling it in size " (Fig. 31, D, Part 1). The vein may bulk still larger.

Section of the clavicle allows rotation of the scapula, which brings structures of axilla *forwards*, and, notably, the deep-seated circumflex nerve.

Before proceeding to the neck let us improve acquaintance with the *layers* of cervical fascia and (like an expert " digging up the past ") enlist their help as guides.

THE DEEP FASCIAL PLANES ABOVE THE CLAVICLE

Three are found here. The first is an *investing layer* which gives a sheath to trapezius and sternomastoid, and cloaks the

---

[1] By this I do not mean the futile thing, of late in regular supply, which cut slowly and broke quickly—even with careful punctilio in the matter of angulation. I mean the tough Gigli saws (chosen with characteristic flair) that form part of the neurosurgeon's armoury. They cost a trifle more ; they cut fast, and for two years I watched class after class bend them double and pass them on intact.

[2] ' Transverse scapular ' (B.N.A.): a factitious, ' portmanteau ' title caught from the well-named transverse cervical vessels that lie contagiously. ' Transverse ' they certainly are—in the neck ; ' scapular ', certainly in destination. But certainly not ' transverse scapular ' : they have a lengthwise course along the bone.

intervening triangle. Deep to this layer is a mass of fat and glands mingled with terminal twigs of transverse cervical and supra-scapular vessels.

Next comes a loose, *intermediate layer* of deep fascia which loops round the posterior belly of omohyoid and, like a mesentery,

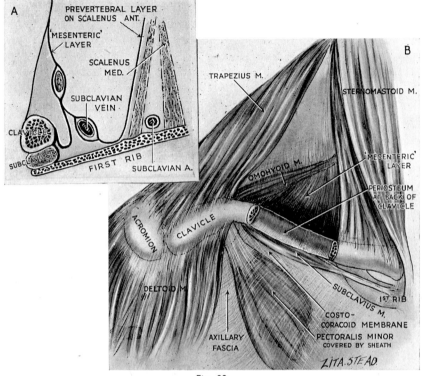

Fig. 32

The three planes of deep fascia above the clavicle. The diagram A (after Paulet) shows the three layers in sagittal section. Note how the ' mesenteric ' layer, which contains the omohyoid, dips behind the clavicle. B shows the continuity of the ' mesenteric ' layer— through the medium of the clavicular periosteum—with the sheath of subclavius (as seen in A), and thence with costocoracoid membrane, and sheath of pectoralis minor.

holds the muscle to the back of clavicle. Here the fascia blends with periosteum through which it is continuous with the hinder layer of subclavius sheath, and that descends towards the chest to form the costocoracoid membrane which gives a covering to pectoralis minor (Fig. 32).[1]

It will thus be clear that when we divide the clavicle we open

[1] My appreciation of a fibrous sheet spreading (beyond both) from omohyoid to pectoralis minor, and crossed but not broken by the adhering clavicle, is due to an admirable specimen made by my friend, Major E. E. Dunlop, D.A.D.M.S., Royal Australian Army Medical Corps.

this second, ' mesenteric ' layer—unless, of course, we first shell
the bone out of its periosteum. The omohyoid belly may lie far
down, behind the clavicle, or rise some fingerbreadths above it
on a long ' mesentery ' ; it is a guide of great worth—a bathymetric
muscle that measures the *depth* we have attained—and (like the
posterior belly of digastric) flags the subjacent presence of all the
neurovascular structures of chief account in its own part of the
neck. Deep to the ' mesenteric ' layer is a second complex of fat
and glands, containing this time the main trunks of the transverse
cervical and suprascapular vessels.

The third and last layer of deep fascia is the *prevertebral* ; it
spreads like a tight sheath of dull cellophane over the front of the
scalene mass, binding on to these muscles the mesh of brachial
plexus, the subclavian artery, and the phrenic nerve. Under this
layer there is *no* mass of fat and glands.[1] (It will be noticed that
mention has not been made of the subclavian vein which lies sunk
in this region, divorced from its artery by scalenus anterior. It
is closely bound to the innermost part of the clavicle but is far
enough away at the point of section to be avoided easily by
hugging the bone.)

THE CERVICAL EXPOSURE RESUMED.—With these facts grasped
we may proceed in all confidence, recognising and dealing with
each stratum in turn—the three fascial layers ; the two fatty
screens. We shall divulse the fat and spare the vascular twigs
by means of Mayo scissors, opening the fascial layers with the same
respect we have for peritoneum, or—in the case of the last layer,
the prevertebral—for dura mater ; and with no less assurance.
(The belly of the omohyoid may be severed or drawn aside, as is
convenient.)

THE MEDIAL EXTENSION THROUGH STERNOMASTOID.—Should we
wish to carry our exposure in across the neck, we must divide the
clavicular head of sternomastoid—an act that calls for circumspec-
tion : the internal jugular vein is often fixed in fat to the deep face
of the muscle. Old periadenitis—as over the carotid fork—may
felt the structures too closely for ' blunt ' separation, making it
most dangerous to slide a finger under and pick up this head of

---

[1] *Deep juxtaclavicular fascial layers of neck.*—These three may be remembered as layers
in a club sandwich arranged thus : (1) *investing layer of deep fascia* ; (2) complex of fat,
glands, and terminal twigs of transverse cervical and suprascapular vessels ; (3) *intermediate* (' *mesenteric* ') *layer of deep fascia* enclosing the posterior belly of omohyoid ;
(4) complex of fat, glands, main branches and tributaries of transverse cervical and
suprascapular vessels ; (5) *prevertebral* (' *cellophane* ') *layer of deep fascia*.

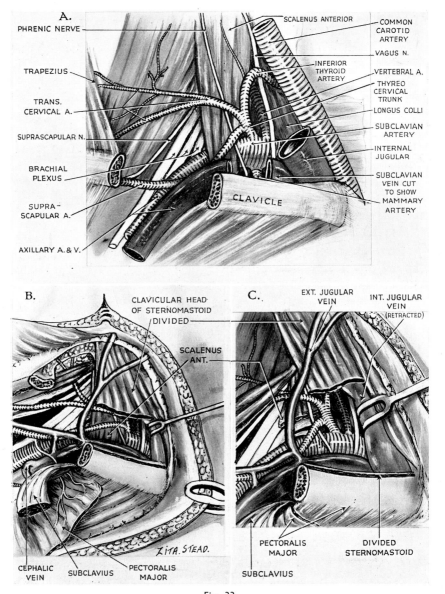

Fig. 33

The axillo-cervical exposure extended medially

The upper figure, A, is to remind us of anatomy. Sternomastoid has been entirely removed.   B. Divide the clavicular head of sternomastoid *surgically* (see text), respecting external and internal jugular veins ; scalenus comes to view. Isolate scalenus *as you would an artery*, releasing phrenic nerve and vessels crossing it.   C. Divide scalenus near the first rib.   Note that its costal end withdraws and lets the two subclavian trunks touch in their second stage. Note how the lowest trunk of brachial plexus is ensconced between scalenus medius and subclavian artery.   The posterior belly of omohyoid is not labelled in B and C.   In B it is partly hidden by the distal piece of clavicle whose cut face shows how the weight of the limb has rotated the shoulder girdle.
     (Clavicle, as a rule, hides the subclavian vein ; here the vein is high.)

sternomastoid for mass division. It is wiser, therefore (after dividing the ' safe ' lateral fingerbreadth), to cut gradually through the front of the head, and use a finger to displace the deepest fibres from the vein.

The subclavian artery in continuity.—Section of the clavicular head of sternomastoid gives a good view of scalenus anterior with a glimpse of phrenic nerve (still under its cellophane fascia) sloping down and in across the muscle. Then, if we first free the nerve and its small companion vessels, we can isolate the scalene muscle as we should isolate a great longitudinal artery ; and after cutting through the belly close above the rib all three stages of subclavian trunk are seen in continuity (Fig. 33, c). Most of the branches, too, are visible, or can be brought to light by gentle blunt dissection. The vertebral artery with the vein in front of it disappears up into the apex of the deep angular space between the divided scalene muscle and the longus colli clothing the vertebral column. (Fig. 33, A, shows the origins of subclavian branches. Note the thyreocervical trunk rising and branching beside the inner scalene edge, directly opposite internal mammary.)

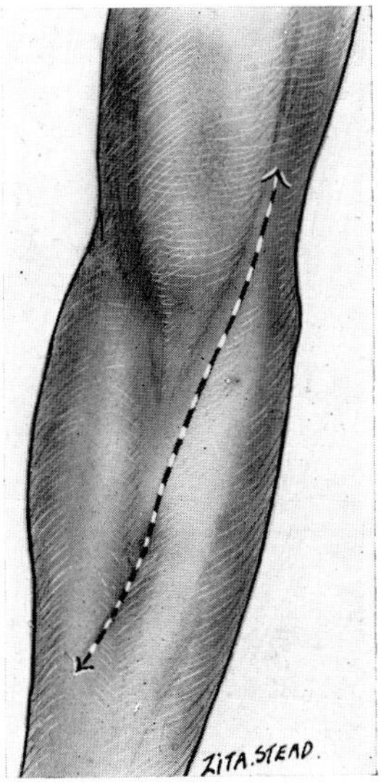

THE DISTAL PART OF THE HUMERUS EXPOSED IN CONTINUITY WITH ANTECUBITAL STRUCTURES

What follows is a mere variant of the innocuous and beautiful exposure described by Fiolle and Delmas, which brings to light the least accessible part of the ulnar vessels and median nerve, and I shall first indicate their method. A skin incision medial to the biceps goes down beside the tendon, and then obliquely out to the junction of the lower and middle thirds of radius ; nothing is cut except skin, superficial fascia and veins. The deep fascia is carefully opened.

Fig. 34

Showing how the biceps tendon dips into the antecubital V

Beside and medial to biceps is the Fiolle and Delmas incision ; it is designed solely for neurovascular structures. In order to expose these structures *in company with humerus* (and elbow joint) the upper part of our incision lies *lateral* to biceps (see Fig. 35, A).

In this region the biceps tendon dips into the wide part of a muscular V (Fig. 34), whose medial limb is the pronator teres flanked by flexor muscles ; the lateral limb of the V is the brachio-

4

radialis with two other bellies that form a wad which can be grasped and moved below the elbow (p. 53). After dividing the tight surrounding sleeve of fascia the two limbs of the V part easily ; if then the forearm is flexed and placed in full pronation, the muscles covering deep-lying ' difficult ' portions of ulnar vessels and median nerve relax and give wide access to every antecubital structure.

Remembering this method we combine exposure of the humerus with easy exploration of the fossa, although the upper part of our incision is on the *outer* side of biceps and therefore opposite to that of Fiolle and Delmas.

THE OPERATION

With the patient's elbow extended and the forearm supine continue the lateral incision for the shaft of humerus (p. 32) beyond the antecubital fossa, curving it out to end two-thirds of the way down the radius (Fig. 35). When we reflect the skin covering the tendon of biceps we shall find the stout band of bicipital fascia (lacertus fibrosus) that forms a sort of retinaculum over the median nerve and distal end of the brachial artery. Dividing the band we then proceed to rip the sleeve of fascia that constricts the ante-cubital V and cramps its limbs together. But once these limbs are free, a finger, dipping in between, can easily disrupt the loose connecting tissues which " break and disappear like soap-suds."

Find the origins of the radial and ulnar arteries close to the inner side of the biceps tendon. Look for the median nerve still farther in beyond them. Mobilise these neurovascular structures by gently opening Mayo scissors close alongside ; then put the forearm into full pronation and draw the limbs of the V apart. The whole complexion of the wound is suddenly transformed : a beggarly view becomes a wide prospect with every structure fortunately placed (Fig. 35, B).

The interosseous artery and its anterior interosseous branch.— These wide and deeply situated branches are hidden underneath a double screen : the parent ulnar trunk lies on their origin, and it is masked in turn by the main radial vessels. These last are mobilised by cutting twigs that moor them to the muscles. A fan-like set (called ' radial recurrent ' from *upper* twigs that loop towards the elbow) is found at once : a finger moving down the outer face of biceps tendon will catch the loop and let us cut the fan. Then forceps on the severed stem rotate the radial artery and veins

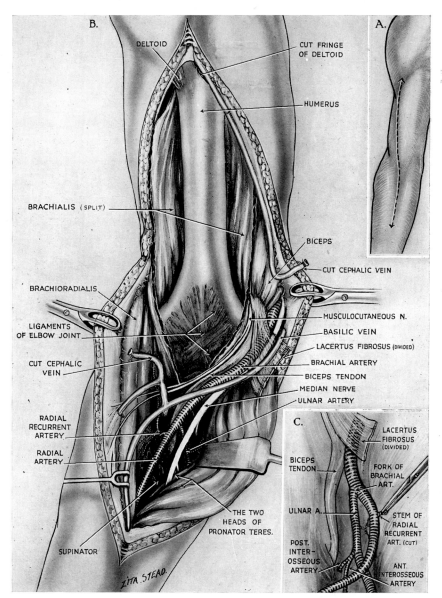

Fig. 35

Extension of distal humeral exposure to the antecubital fossa

A. The whole incision. This is made with the limb supine. B. The exposure. The forearm is now *pronated*, relaxing the antecubital V so that retraction shows the deep part of the ulnar artery. C. Division of the stem of the vascular fan formed by the so-called ' radial recurrent' provides a handle for rotation and displacement of the brachial fork towards the ulnar shaft—a movement which uncovers interosseous vessels.

away towards the ulnar shaft, uncovering the ulnar artery and drawing it aside by gentle force transmitted through the parent brachial trunk (Fig. 35, c).

This simple movement inwards of radial and ulnar affords a full exposure of our interosseous objectives and yields a thorough view of veins and arteries that ramify within the fossa—a place whose depths should cease to give excuse for hæmostatic rooting.

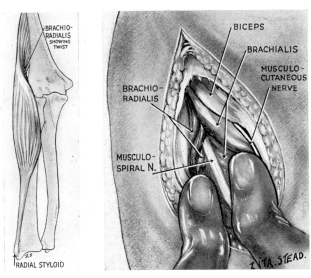

Fig. 36

Finding the distal end of the musculospiral (radial) nerve

A thumb on each muscle opens the spiral plane of cleavage between brachioradialis and brachialis as one would open a book. Inset, The twist of brachioradialis which is moulded to the tapering brachialis.

FINDING THE DISTAL END OF THE MUSCULOSPIRAL (OR RADIAL) NERVE.—There is sometimes delay in finding this part of the nerve. It lies here in a peculiar *spiral* plane of cleavage between brachioradialis on the lateral side and brachialis on the medial; for where these bellies touch the brachialis tapers while its fellow twists. So, after dividing deep fascia do not use a knife to reach the nerve; instead place well-gloved thumbs, lengthwise and parallel, one on each belly, and open the plane—like a book on your knee. The nerve marks the place (Fig. 36).

THE FRONT OF THE FOREARM

ANATOMY

We shall consider the muscles first; their arrangement in respect of each other, and sometimes their intimate constitution, are clues to several exposures. So we shall make it easy for the mind to build the part like a model—and then take it to bits.

The mobile wad of three.—Let us first exclude three muscles we have met already (p. 50), which can be grasped with finger and thumb, and moved to and fro as a mobile wad just below the lateral epicondyle of the humerus (Fig. 37). They are, from before back, brachioradialis, and the long and short radial extensors of the wrist. These mobile bellies flank the radius on the outer side and ride at anchor on a fan-shaped leash of vessels from the radial trunks—a leash we must divide before we can retract the muscles outwards or the trunks in (pp. 50, 58).

The rest.—The remaining muscles are arranged as three groups : (1) superficial ; (2) intermediate ; (3) deep.

The *superficial group* consists of four muscles, remembered by placing the *ball* of the opposite thumb on the front of the medial epicondyle, letting the thumb and *three* fingers point along the supine forearm (Fig. 38). The thumb lies obliquely and marks the course of the oblique pronator teres ; the index finger touches the tendon of flexor carpi radialis close by the radial pulse ; the middle finger takes the place of a frequent absentee—palmaris longus ; the ring finger covers the last muscle

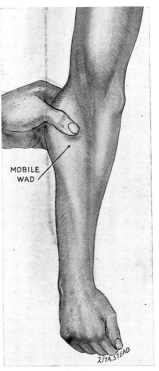

MOBILE WAD

Fig. 37

Recognition of the mobile wad of three muscles below the lateral epicondyle of humerus

The muscles, from before back, are brachioradialis, long and short radial extensors. This wad can be moved *across* the part of radius clothed by supinator, *against* the neighbouring muscles. The anterior and posterior edges of the wad, defined in this way, serve as guides for making incisions and discovering planes of cleavage (see Figs. 45 and 57, A).

53

of the group, flexor carpi ulnaris. (The little finger plays no part

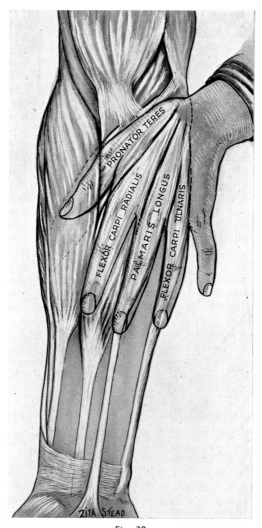

Fig. 38

**A manual mnemonic for superficial muscles
on the front of the forearm**

Place the opposite hand on the front of the forearm
as in the figure, with the thenar eminence covering
the medial epicondyle. Thumb and fingers indicate
the lie of superficial muscles ; the little finger plays
no part. Note how pronator makes a bridge across
the forearm.

in these manual mnemonics which we shall do well to practise first
on our own forearms.)

The *intermediate group* has one muscle only—flexor digitorum sublimis—but a muscle of some complexity, whose close and peculiar relations with the median nerve are of practical importance. Its tendons go under the transverse carpal ligament as if they had ' formed two deep '—a fact which betokens the two-layered arrangement of the fleshy parts. The *superficial portion* of sublimis belonging to the front-rank tendons—for ring and middle finger—is a thin sheet that slants across from humerus to radius bridging the interval between the bones of the forearm (Fig. 39). The median nerve and the deep, ' difficult ' portions of the ulnar vessels diverge as they leave the antecubital fossa and pass beneath this bridge, whose arch—which gives them entry—has varying relations with the bridging belly of pronator teres. Pronator either overspreads the

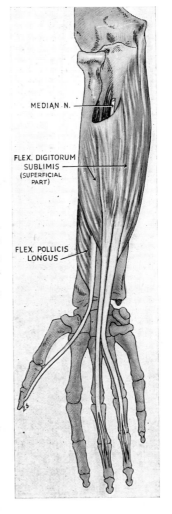

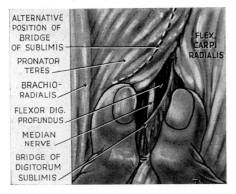

MEDIAN N.

FLEX. DIGITORUM SUBLIMIS (SUPERFICIAL PART)

FLEX. POLLICIS LONGUS

ALTERNATIVE POSITION OF BRIDGE OF SUBLIMIS

FLEX. CARPI RADIALIS

PRONATOR TERES

BRACHIO-RADIALIS

FLEXOR DIG. PROFUNDUS

MEDIAN NERVE

BRIDGE OF DIGITORUM SUBLIMIS

Fig. 39

The superficial part of sublimis

This part gives rise to the two front-rank tendons (for ring and middle finger). It forms a bridge whose oblique entrance may have a high or low level in the forearm and thus be either deep or distal to pronator teres. The median nerve therefore runs either under a two-layered arch (formed by pronator plus sublimis), or else must cross a gap between two separate spans. (See inset where flexor carpi radialis has been retracted to show the median in the gap. The dotted line indicates the proximal variety of sublimis arch.)

arch of the sublimis (forming a double-layered span), or else sublimis lies more distally (so that the spans are separated by a gap)—a point of some importance in looking for the median nerve (p. 65).

The *deep part of sublimis* is trigastric (Fig. 40) ; the two distal bellies correspond to the rear-rank tendons—for index and little

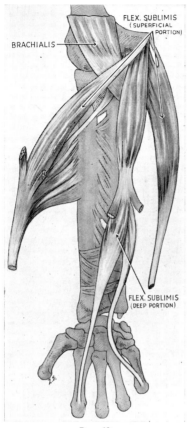

Fig. 40
**The deep part of sublimis
(after Poirier)**

The two distal bellies of the trigastric portion give tendons to little finger and index—the rear-rank tendons which enter the wrist behind those of the other two fingers. The median nerve is bound in satellite relation to the radial side of the deep part of sublimis.

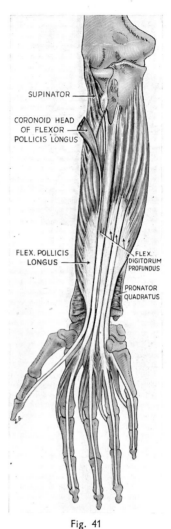

Fig. 41
**The deep anterior muscles
met in surgical exposure**

One lies lengthwise along each bone. One joins the proximal ends of the bones, one the distal.

finger ; the proximal belly springs from the common origin on the medial epicondyle of the humerus.

The satellite median.—After leaving the antecubital space the median nerve becomes a satellite of the deep part of sublimis, lying first to the radial side of the proximal belly ; then to the radial side of the intermediate tendon which is sometimes an obvious glistening thing, but often dull and cord-like enough to simulate the nerve itself. Below this level, fascia binds the median

in a lateral groove between the front- and rear-rank tendons that go respectively to middle and index fingers. The nerve, therefore, stays with sublimis if we separate that muscle from profundus. We shall see (on p. 68) how to find the median near the wrist.

Loose tissue joins the single, intermediate, sublimis to the deep group, forming a plane of facile cleavage that is used with great advantage by McConnell (p. 66).

The *deep anterior group* consists of four muscles (Fig. 41): one lies along the length of each bone —the flexor of the thumb upon the radius, profundus digitorum on the ulna. The other muscles cross *between* the bones — the supinator near the elbow, the flat quadratus near the wrist. (I know I contravene morphology by classing supinator with anterior muscles, but here we meet the supinator first in *front*; and this book deals in practice.) Note that the tendons of profundus digitorum— unlike the tendons of sublimis—lie in a single rank of four abreast.

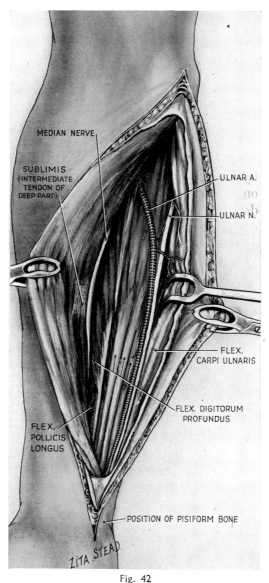

MEDIAN NERVE

SUBLIMIS
(INTERMEDIATE
TENDON OF
DEEP PART)

ULNAR A.

ULNAR N.

FLEX.
CARPI ULNARIS

FLEX. DIGITORUM
PROFUNDUS

FLEX.
POLLICIS
LONGUS

POSITION OF PISIFORM BONE

ZITA STEAD

Fig. 42

The ulnar neurovascular bundle belongs to the *deep* layer of muscles. Note how the bundle splits proximally. The median nerve sticks to sublimis.

The *ulnar nerve* comes to the front of forearm from behind the elbow. It is thus natural to find it fastened to a member of the *deep* group of forearm muscles—flexor digitorum profundus.

The *ulnar vessels* join the nerve at a sharp angle and then go down its radial side, forming a neurovascular bundle (Fig. 42) partitioned from the inner flank of forearm by the tendon of flexor carpi ulnaris. We have already noticed these vessels leaving the antecubital fossa (p. 55); we now see they do so by passing between the deep and intermediate groups of muscle.

The *radial artery* begins at the medial side of the biceps tendon; and so its oblique proximal part becomes a satellite of the oblique pronator teres which also has a medial origin : the artery is bound by fascia to the muscle,[1] though books omit the fact and harp instead on the relation here of brachioradialis. That is why one sees despairing *outward* hunts in the proximal third of forearm to find a vessel which comes from the inner side. This artery, with its companion veins, is dangerously near the surface and may be slit in opening the fascial sleeve of swollen limbs.

The *tendon of biceps* is a major landmark, a vertical partition which divides the proximal portion of the antecubital V into a ' dangerous ' area on the medial side, a ' safe ' one on the lateral —provided of course the knife stays close to the tendon and does not wander out to threaten the end of the musculospiral nerve, the radial of Basle nomenclature.

The tendon leads through loose fat to the tuberosity of radius, a part of which is covered by the *bicipital bursa*—whose aid we shall enlist.

The radial leash, called " recurrent."—Crossing the ' safe ' lateral area of the antecubital fossa is a group of vessels called recurrent radial ; only the most proximal deserve the name by running up the limb ; the other members are important muscular twigs which spread out fanwise to the mobile wad of bellies that flank the radius (p. 50). The wad therefore is moored to the radial trunks by a fan-like vascular leash whose vessels—which rib the fan (Fig. 43)— seldom lie in a single plane but diverge in a set of layers two or three deep ; *all* these must be divided to free the tethered muscles —unless we cut the stem from which they spread. A finger moving

---

[1] The only reference I found to this was not in any standard work but in a small *précis*, owned once by a ward-sister who remembered Bland-Sutton as " a shy young student."

The words in Paulet's book are in italics : " *Il ne faut pas oublier que l'artère radiale n'est pas dans la gaine du long supinateur,*"—the brachioradialis—" *mais dans celle du rond pronateur.*" (V. Paulet, 1884, *Résumé d' Anatomie Appliquée*, Paris, 3 ème Edn., p. 418.)

distally along the outer face of biceps tendon will feel the leash (which lies invisible in fat) and hook it up—a welcome guide in featureless surroundings.

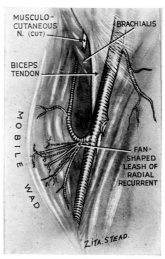

The branch once called the radial branch of musculospiral, alias (in B.N.A.) the superficial terminal branch of radial, and now (in fitful text-books) lumped with the parent stem as ' radial '[1]—this branch, by any name you choose, clings to the mobile wad of muscles, the hinder one of which it may supply.[2] The satellite relation of the nerve and wad involves reciprocal divorce (and therefore easy severance) from close-adjoining radial vessels, which go for their part with pronator teres and then with flexor longus pollicis. (A way of finding the distal end of the parent trunk is described on p. 52.)

The *medial cutaneous nerve* of the forearm lies to the ulnar side of any elective incision we shall make on the front of the limb—excepting McConnell's (p. 66).

Fig. 43

The fan-like leash of vessels called ' radial recurrent '

(The veins are not shown.) Only the proximal rib of the fan is recurrent. The ribs are in several layers—two, three, or four deep. They are muscular branches which tie the mobile wad to the radial vessels.

EXPOSURE OF THE WHOLE SHAFT OF RADIUS FROM IN FRONT WITH EXTENSIONS TO MEDIAN AND ULNAR NERVES

We have thus built a rough but working model of the front of forearm. Let us now take this apart sufficiently to see the whole length of radius.

First, we must still further mobilise the wad of three mobile muscles (brachioradialis, long and short radial wrist-extensors) so that we can draw them well away from the lateral face of radial shaft. We shall therefore use an incision that follows these muscles

[1] Impatient persons (like the *Queen of Hearts*) wish off the heads of *all* who are responsible. But *Alice* (duly coached and kindlier) might put our three nomenclatures in one portmanteau and call the slithy nerve the *radial branch of musculoradial*. (Its deeper fellow is, of course, the *muscular*.)

[2] C. R. Salsbury, *British Journal of Surgery*, 1938, 26, 95.

right into the *arm*. Then, after opening deep fascia, we shall cut the fan-shaped vascular leash—the so-called radial recurrent—which holds them tethered to the main radial trunk. Lastly, we undo the supinator, the deep muscle that comes across from ulna to grasp—like fingers of a hand—the upper third of radial shaft.

The *posterior interosseous nerve* (deep terminal branch of

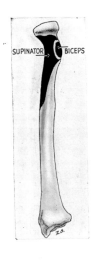 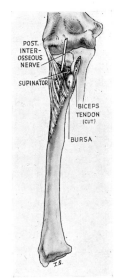

Fig. 44

Anatomical relationships at the upper part of the radius. The white crescent between the two black areas of attachment marks the site of the bicipital bursa and shows how it lies in a bay formed by the supinator edge. The surgeon is guided to the bursa —and thus to the edge of the supinator —by the outer face of the biceps tendon (see insets to Figs. 47 and 48).

radial, B.N.A.) penetrates the anterolateral face of the supinator muscle, and separates its two layers; the deeper layer fends the nerve from radius. The part of supinator edge that skirts the tuberosity of radius curves also round a bursa of the biceps, which lies next bone and lubricates the tendon (Fig. 44). At first loose fat swamps everything; but once we find and cut the fan-shaped leash the outer face of biceps tendon leads us to the bursa, which we divide to reach the tuberosity, thus leaving the rugine a place to come in contact

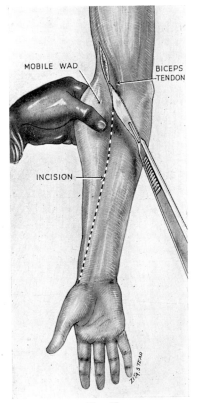

Fig. 45

Incision for anterior exposure of the radius

The knife follows the front edge of the mobile wad (brachioradialis, long and short radial wrist extensors).

with the bone. Then, starting at the *edge* of supinator, we find the muscle easy to detach.

THE OPERATION

Incision.—First, with the limb supine, feel out the mobile wad of three muscles and draw the knife along its medial edge (Fig. 45).

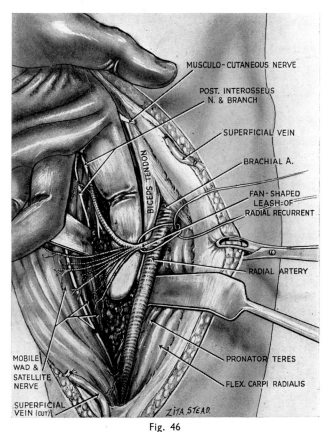

Fig. 46

Finding the fan-like leash

A finger slid lengthwise down the outer side of the biceps tendon feels the resistant loop of the recurrent proximal vessels. Be sure to catch up *all* the layers of the fan—two, three, or four—unless, as in the figure, you tie and cut instead the short single stem of the fan. Note that the radial branch of musculospiral (=superficial terminal branch of radial) is bound in satellite relation to the mobile wad.

The incision goes up a handbreadth into the arm, keeping a finger-breadth lateral to the edge of biceps (see p. 27); below, it reaches to the radial styloid. Divide and tie the large superficial vein that crosses the mid-third of radius, and may continue thence as the cephalic.

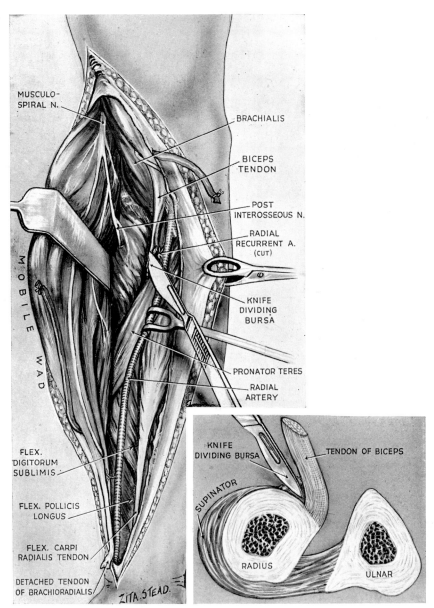

MUSCULO-
SPIRAL N.

BRACHIALIS

BICEPS
TENDON

POST
INTEROSSEOUS N.

RADIAL
RECURRENT A.
(CUT)

KNIFE
DIVIDING
BURSA

M O B I L E   W A D

PRONATOR TERES

RADIAL
ARTERY

KNIFE
DIVIDING BURSA

TENDON OF BICEPS

SUPINATOR

FLEX.
DIGITORUM
SUBLIMIS

FLEX. POLLICIS
LONGUS

FLEX. CARPI
RADIALIS TENDON

DETACHED TENDON
OF BRACHIORADIALIS

RADIUS

ULNAR

ZITA.STEAD.

Fig. 47

The fan-like leash has been cut ; the mobile wad is free for lateral retraction. The knife, with the flat of its blade touching the ' safe ' outer face of biceps tendon, cuts through loose fat ; it then cuts through the bicipital bursa to strike the tuberosity of radius at the edge of the supinator insertion (see inset).

In this figure and the next, two points should be noted : (1) Fat which veils the front of supinator is omitted in order to show the muscle. (In spite of fat the *lining* of the bursal sac will glint when once the knife has cut into the cavity.) (2) The peculiar *distal* course of the cutaneous part of the musculocutaneous nerve is due to its retraction inwards with the skin. Note how the proximal part of the nerve appears at the junction of biceps tendon with biceps belly—a sure guide to its discovery.

The deep guide.—First expose the biceps tendon by dividing deep fascia on its lateral side. Go on dividing this fascia throughout the wound with blunt-nosed scissors, taking special care of the radial vessels. Pass the finger down through the swamp of fat, along the outer side of the guiding tendon till you meet the resistance of the recurrent vascular loop (Fig. 46). Remember that this loop is only the proximal rib of a fan-like spread of vessels that lie in several layers. Hook up *all* the layers of the fan gently on the

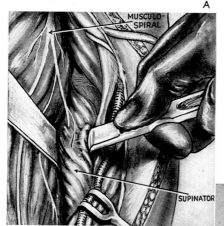

finger; divide and tie them —or tie instead their narrow stem. Mobilise the wad of three long muscles which flanks the outer face of forearm. Detach the flat tendon of brachioradialis from its hold on the base of the radial styloid. Flex the elbow, through 90 degrees

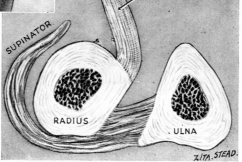

Fig. 48

The rugine working outwards from the site of the divided bursa begins to peel the grasp of supinator from the radial shaft.

and retract the outer muscles widely to expose the supinator.

Return then to the biceps tendon. First make the tendon taut; then, keeping the flat of the knife close to its outer face, cut down upon the bone. The knife divides bicipital bursa, and strikes the tuberosity of radius, which lies embraced within a bay formed by the supinator edge (Fig. 47). From this strategic point the rugine peels the supinator muscle off the bone (Fig. 48). The muscle is turned outwards, sandwiching within its substance the posterior interosseous nerve (deep terminal branch of radial, B.N.A.).

Lastly, a vital part of the exposure: put the forearm into full pronation; the radius then will be revealed from end to end (Fig. 49).

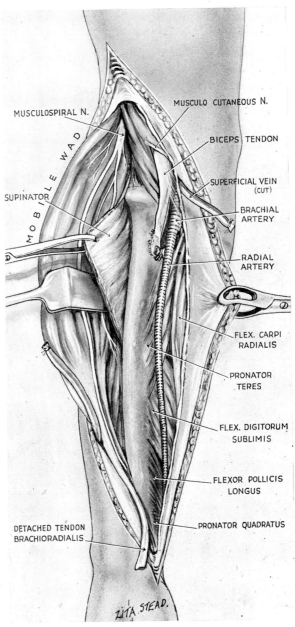

MUSCULOSPIRAL N.

MUSCULO CUTANEOUS N.

MOBILE WAD

BICEPS TENDON

SUPINATOR

SUPERFICIAL VEIN
(CUT)

BRACHIAL
ARTERY

RADIAL
ARTERY

FLEX. CARPI
RADIALIS

PRONATOR
TERES

FLEX. DIGITORUM
SUBLIMIS

FLEXOR POLLICIS
LONGUS

PRONATOR QUADRATUS

DETACHED TENDON
BRACHIORADIALIS

ZITA STEAD.

Fig. 49

The forearm remains supine till supinator is mobilised.
Complete the exposure by putting the forearm into full
pronation ; this will bring the bone to the surface, as in the
figure.

UNREDUCED ANTERIOR LUXATIONS OF THE RADIAL HEAD.— These injuries are common where men fight with quarterstaffs. A forearm guards the skull from a descending blow whose force, breaking the ulna, drives the fragments on against the radius and thrusts its head in front. Then, if a closed reduction fails, the upper third of the complete exposure will serve for reposition or resection.

EXTENDING THE EXPOSURE OF RADIUS TO THE MEDIAN AND ULNAR NERVES.—Should we wish to extend the exposure, we have already seen how this is done for nerves and vessels of the antecubital region (p. 49): an attack begun there from the outer side of humerus was carried over to include them all. Let us now with equal ease spread our exposure of the radial shaft to embrace the median and ulnar nerves in the rest of the forearm—the distal two-thirds. If we begin our approach to the bone with a view to including these nerves, we shall of course make the forearm-portion of the incision nearer the middle line than if radius were our sole objective; though in any forearm a *long* incision combined with trivial skin-reflection will bring us where we wish.

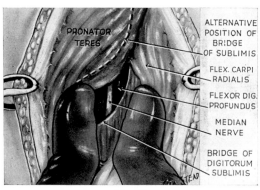

Fig. 50

Finding the median nerve distal to pronator teres. —Begin to separate the belly of pronator teres from that of flexor carpi radialis *where they diverge.* Use the thumbs back to back to move the muscles harmlessly apart. A short length of median *may* appear between pronator and sublimis, as in this figure. If not, you must split the thin superficial part of sublimis to see the nerve.

Exposing the median nerve from in front.—We must first find the plane of cleavage between pronator teres and flexor carpi radialis (between thumb and index of the manual mnemonic in Fig. 38). The *tendons* of these two muscles separate widely in the distal third of forearm, the place, of course, from which to prise apart the close-packed bellies—a thing most gently done with two thumbs back to back (Fig. 50). And now a short, flat-looking piece of median trunk will often show in the proximal part of the separation; it goes between the distal edge of pronator and the proximal edge of the bridge-like portion of sublimis. This glimpse of nerve (Fig. 50) is only possible when the sublimis bridge lies

5

farther down the limb than the more superficial span of pronator teres—leaving a gap for the nerve to cross (p. 55). But when one span lies level with the other and covers it, there is no gap nor glimpse at all : there is instead (between our separating thumbs) an unrevealing face—the thin bridge of sublimis, whose grain we now must split to see the nerve. We know already we shall find it bound by a transparent fascia to the deep, trigastric part of that two-layered muscle.

The ulnar nerve exposed from in front.—If we wish to include the ulnar in the anterior approach, we must open the plane between sublimis and the deep layer, relaxing sublimis by flexing the hand and drawing the muscle forwards. We shall then see that the space is closed on the ulnar side by a shining band of tendon, the flexor carpi ulnaris ; beside it we shall find the ulnar nerve—bound, with the vessels, to deep flexor digitorum. Combined exposure of median and ulnar nerves is thus obtained as a by-product of the approach to radial shaft.

But, if our quarry in the forearm happens to be the distal two-thirds of median nerve, or the whole length of ulnar nerve—or both ; or if a *medial* wound determines our direction, then we can make use of an exposure that has the " simple elegance " which Horace praised, joined (this time) with fidelity.

McCONNELL'S COMBINED EXPOSURE OF MEDIAN AND ULNAR NERVES IN THE FOREARM [1]

Lay the forearm supine. Incise skin only—from *radial* edge of pisiform to medial epicondyle (Fig. 51). Open deep fascia along the radial side of flexor carpi ulnaris tendon, working up from the distal end of the wound. The ulnar nerve and vessels are found at once and traced in a proximal direction to the sharp angle where they part company, the line of the vessels turning outwards from the straight course of the nerve (Fig. 51). It is then easy to find the friendly plane of cleavage between sublimis mass and flexor profundus (Fig. 52). The median nerve, we know, lies, in a shallow groove, upon sublimis, to the radial side of its deep trigastric portion. So, when the plane is opened up, nerve and sublimis move (and stay) in company.

It is often easy to mistake the intermediate tendon of the deep, trigastric moiety for the median nerve (Fig. 51), and I shall

[1] A. A. McConnell, *Dublin Journal of Medical Science*, 1920, p. 90.

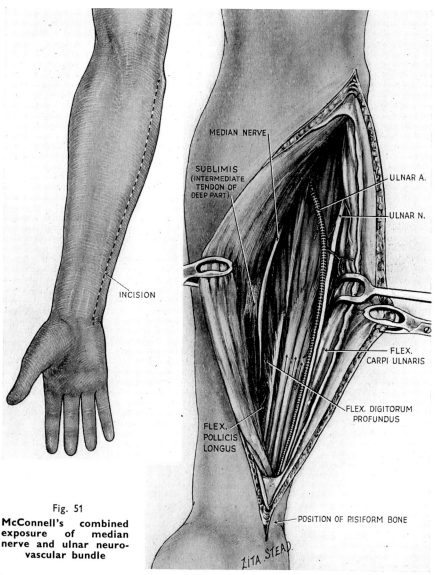

MEDIAN NERVE

SUBLIMIS
(INTERMEDIATE
TENDON OF
DEEP PART)

ULNAR A.

ULNAR N.

INCISION

FLEX.
CARPI ULNARIS

FLEX. DIGITORUM
PROFUNDUS

FLEX.
POLLICIS
LONGUS

POSITION OF PISIFORM BONE

ZITA STEAD.

Fig. 51

**McConnell's combined
exposure of median
nerve and ulnar neuro-
vascular bundle**

Incision runs from medial epicondyle to pisiform. The plane between sublimis and profundus
is opened up. Note how the median sticks to the sublimis 'roof'; the ulnar bundle sticks
to the profundus 'floor.' Note, too, the intermediate tendon which sometimes simulates
the median.

close with a double counsel : Do not too quickly rejoice at the first cord-like structure you may see—it is possibly a flexor tendon ; do not cut into the deep face of sublimis to look for the nerve ; you will only make a mess.

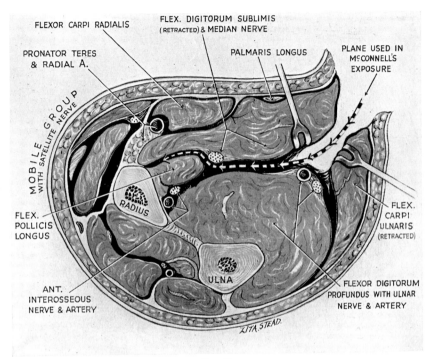

Fig. 52

Cross-section showing the plane of cleavage in McConnell's exposure

The plane is entered in front of flexor carpi ulnaris and in front of the ulnar bundle ; it lies between the intermediate layer of muscle (which consists only of sublimis) and the deep layer. The median nerve sticks to the ' roof ' ; the ulnar bundle to the ' floor.' (In practice entry is effected at a more distal and facile level—in front of the *tendon* of flexor carpi ulnaris.)

EXPOSURE OF THE MEDIAN NERVE ABOVE THE WRIST

The nerve just here is literally median, a fact to grasp if we would find it quickly ; for, despite tradition, palmaris longus is a mere decoy and has no value as a landmark. Out of 100 forearms, Tandler (that attractive person whose good work embraced both quick and dead) notes how the median lay behind or radial to palmaris tendon in 53 ; in 35, the nerve lay to its inner side ; in 12 he found no tendon. And I would add that when the median does lie close behind palmaris, the tendon often moves away once we retract deep fascia.

Other relations near the wrist.—The nerve—true satellite of the sublimis mass—keeps on one level and so comes near the surface at the wrist ; for the limb tapers as the bellies shrink, leaving the nerve bare of flesh and flanked by tendon. But even here the inner edge of median (still faithful to sublimis) weds the groove between the front-rank middle finger tendon and its rear-rank index-finger file. The groove is deepened by the pointed fleshy tongues that coat these tendons till they reach the wrist ; and up the groove a severed median may withdraw from sight.

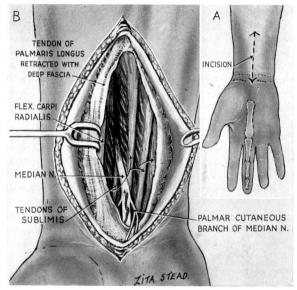

Fig. 53

Exposure of the median nerve close above the wrist

A. The axis-line incision reaching the distal 'bracelet.'
B. The exposure. Palmaris longus is retracted with deep fascia. The *fixed* relation of the nerve is to the middle-finger tendon of sublimis, in front of which it winds.

THE OPERATION

The axis line.—The certain guide (because the nerve is median) is the long axis of the middle metacarpal bone—produced, of course, into the forearm (Fig. 53). So make the knife continue that long axis up the limb. Begin incising at the distal 'bracelet' which marks the forearm skin, and end the cut at least four fingerbreadths above. Use this line, too, for opening the deep fascia ; displace the chance obtrusion of palmaris tendon. The nerve is seen at once, marked often by a small meandering vessel.

Above, the median disappears beneath a pointed fleshy tongue of the sublimis ; below, and near the ' bracelets,' it gives a branch which overlies the parent trunk and goes to palmar skin. The main nerve leaves the wound beneath the bridge of transverse carpal ligament, and, just before it vanishes from sight, lies on the *front* of the sublimis tendon for the middle finger (Fig. 53).

This exposure may, of course, continue, or be continued into, the *anterior* approach to median and ulnar nerves described on p. 65 above.

THE BACK OF THE FOREARM

The arrangement of parts here is very simple.

The *mobile wad* is the same wad of three muscles we know already :—extensors (radial) long and short, brachioradialis—a boring refrain, but useful in practice ; nor should we scorn the metre which comes (with a past) from the very front of the chorus.

These three muscles are moved at will with finger and thumb, not only across the radial shaft (clothed by supinator), but also *against* the neighbouring mass of common extensor that lies more firmly bound. Presently their mobility will help us to find and rip a seam in the cloak covering the neuromuscular sandwich of supinator and posterior interosseous nerve.

The rest of the muscles.—Excluding the mobile wad, the muscles on the back of forearm lie in two layers—superficial and deep. We can now proceed, as we did in front, to make a manual mnemonic for the *surface layer*. But this time we must carry the ball of the opposite thumb round *behind* the forearm and place it on the back of the lateral epicondyle (Fig. 54). The oblique thumb again (but rather awkwardly) marks an oblique muscle—the anconeus. The index will press the belly of extensor carpi ulnaris against the ulnar shaft ; the middle finger marks extensor digiti quinti, while the ring finger lies on the rather fixed mass of common extensor. (The little finger is not used at all.)

The deep layer.—There is good reason to remember the arrangement of this layer (Fig. 55). All its tendons (excepting sometimes that of proprius) can be seen in one's own hand ; all go to thumb or index. They are four in number : abductor pollicis longus, extensor pollicis brevis, extensor pollicis longus, extensor indicis proprius. Except for the first—the long abductor which springs from *both* bones—the tendons point towards their bone of origin.

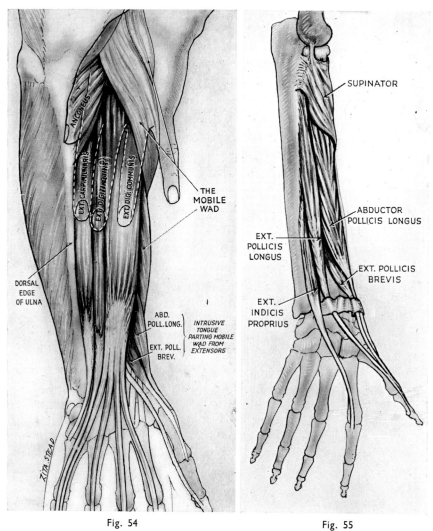

Fig. 54

Manual mnemonic for posterior superficial muscles of the forearm

The ball of the opposite thumb lies this time on the *back* of lateral epicondyle. The index finger feels the dorsal edge of ulnar shaft. (Again the little finger plays no part.)

Fig. 55

The deep posterior muscles

These send their tendons to thumb or index. (Supinator also makes a wide posterior appearance. It has already been described and dealt with in the front of the limb.)

So the short thumb extensor comes from radius; the long extensor and the proprius from ulna. (The bellies of two muscles of the thumb, the long abductor and short extensor, thrust out a common

fleshy tongue between the mobile wad of three and the more fixed
extensor of the fingers—a tongue which
helps to emphasise the parting we shall
presently exploit.) [1]

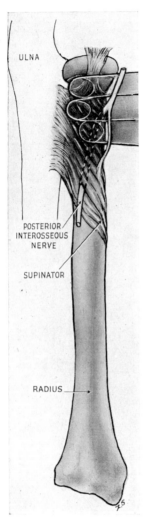

ULNA

POSTERIOR
INTEROSSEOUS
NERVE

SUPINATOR

RADIUS

Fig. 56

The three-finger method
of locating the posterior
interosseous nerve (deep
terminal branch of
musculospiral)

The test must be applied
at the *back* of radius. The
edge of the proximal finger-
tip fits the curve where head
joins neck. Sandwiched in
fibres of supinator, the nerve
crosses the back of radius
deep to the pulp of the
distal finger-tip.

We have seen (p. 60) how the posterior
interosseous nerve (the deep terminal
branch of musculospiral) enters the anterolateral face of supinator and slopes
obliquely down across the striped grain of
that muscle. The nerve can be found on
the *back* of radial shaft at a quite definite
point—three fingerbreadths distal to the
head of radius (Fig. 56). I would stress the
fact that this measurement must be made
neither on the outer side of the bone, nor
on its posterolateral face, but on the back
only.

EXPOSURE OF THE POSTERIOR INTER-
OSSEOUS NERVE (THE DEEP TERMINAL
BRANCH OF THE MUSCULOSPIRAL)
FROM BEHIND

This nerve, they say, is difficult to find.
The fault, however, is not in the *nerve*.
Its faithful rendezvous upon the back of
radius (like that kept by the parent trunk
in skirting round the humerus) is just
another of those ' certainties ' on which it
is unfair to bet.

THE OPERATION

Incision.—The knife should aim to go
between extensor carpi radialis brevis and
extensor digitorum communis (Stookey and

---

[1] The site of separation is further marked by a pit which
can be felt in the *prone* forearm just proximal to the
bulge of the intrusive ' tongue,' a handbreadth above
the wrist. The finger-tip receives a sharp impression of
the shaft of radius, unpadded at the bottom of the pit by
tendon or by belly.

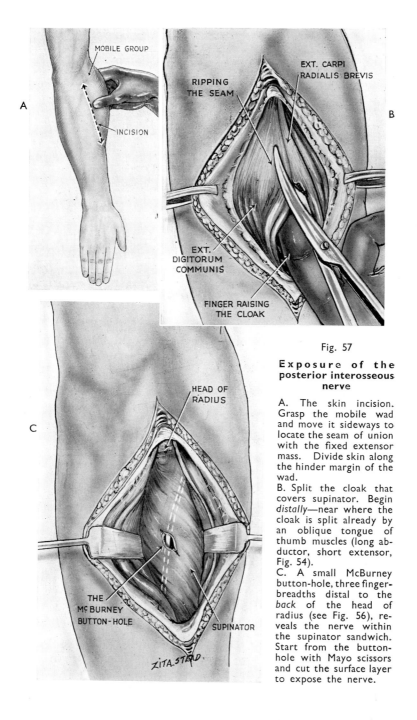

Fig. 57

Exposure of the posterior interosseous nerve

A. The skin incision. Grasp the mobile wad and move it sideways to locate the seam of union with the fixed extensor mass. Divide skin along the hinder margin of the wad.

B. Split the cloak that covers supinator. Begin *distally*—near where the cloak is split already by an oblique tongue of thumb muscles (long abductor, short extensor, Fig. 54).

C. A small McBurney button-hole, three finger-breadths distal to the *back* of the head of radius (see Fig. 56), reveals the nerve within the supinator sandwich. Start from the button-hole with Mayo scissors and cut the surface layer to expose the nerve.

Guild, 1919).[1] With the patient's forearm prone the line for separating these is found at once by grasping with a thumb and finger the wad that lies just distal to the outer epicondyle. This wad (whose hindmost belly *is* extensor carpi radialis brevis) moves readily against the much less mobile mass of the communis. We therefore easily locate the *hinder* margin of the wad and trace it with a knife (at first through skin) a generous handbreadth down the limb, from outer epicondyle (Fig. 57).

When we have opened deep fascia—beginning distally—we verify once more the plane between the zones of different mobility, and take advantage of their distal parting to separate them cleanly. This pair of bellies covers supinator with a loose cloak, ripped easily in two where it divides but toughly fused above within a fibrous hood. A finger, therefore, working from below, will help to raise the cloak for clean division (Fig. 57). Then we shall see the striped (and sometimes flashy) supinator belly. The nerve (sandwiched, remember, in the muscle) slopes *across* the stripe. Measure then with the tips of three fingers—side by side and touching—from the *back* of the neck of radius ; the posterior interosseous nerve lies on the *back* of shaft deep to the distal finger (Fig. 56, above). And here a small McBurney cut, splitting the supinator grain, will let us glimpse the flat and whitish shape of our objective ; and then, if we transect the grain, we shall expose the nerve. A word of caution : the sandwich is *thin*, so do not nick the nerve with your McBurney.

EXPOSURE OF THE HEAD AND NECK
OF RADIUS FROM BEHIND

It has been said that any cut made behind the proximal end of radius will expose the head and neck of the bone safely, provided that it stops before we wound the posterior interosseous nerve. This statement is soundly based : extensor digitorum communis takes origin within a hood of tough fibrous tissue that lies behind the radial head and yields no plane of cleavage. We shall accordingly divide the skin and then cut down on bone, using three fingers to locate the nerve (Fig. 56), and cutting only to the second nail. (The cut should also reach two fingerbreadths *above* the epicondyle to leave room for resection.)

---

[1] S. Guild and B. Stookey, *Surgery, Gynecology and Obstetrics*, 1919, **28,** 612.

TWO EXPOSURES IN THE HAND

A MEDIAL APPROACH TO
MID-PALMAR SPACE AND ULNAR BURSA [1]

Adams McConnell—the first by many years, this side of the Atlantic, to give Kanavel's work a practical appreciation—described in 1913 a method of draining the mid-palmar space (*Medical Press and Circular*, 1913, **95**, 328). His dorsal incision of the web between the fingers, remote alike from vessels, nerves and palmar skin, has not been bettered.[2] It is a part, however, of its charm that surgery leaves room for new alternatives. The one I shall describe gives access to the space and ulnar bursa. Advantage will be taken of a loop-hole in the *edge* of the hand to gain entry to the palm. The skin incision, like McConnell's, leaves no palmar scar, and gives dependent drainage both of space and bursa when the hand lies semi-prone, in its most comfortable attitude.

ANATOMY

The floor of the palm is formed by alternate bones and interosseous muscles covered with a loose carpet of fascia—a carpet separated from the ulnar bursa by mid-palmar space. The bursa wraps the superficial and deep flexor tendons of middle, ring, and little fingers and almost fills the space.[3]

The way in.—Opponens of the little finger, the deepest hypothenar muscle, lies on the ulnar side of palmar floor concealed by the short flexor and the large bulge of abductor. It is fastened proximally to the hook of unciform and to the transverse carpal ligament; distally, to the distal three-quarters of the fifth meta-

---

[1] *The Lancet*, 1939, **1**, 16.

[2] There is, I know, a prejudice abroad which holds that specialists, like cobblers, should stick to their last. And so, in case it were believed by any that the hand of *one* employment " hath the daintier touch," the fact is worth attention that this neurosurgeon was amongst the first (if not the first) to integrate Cushing's technique outside America; certainly first (as Dandy notes) to use ventriculography in Europe. But never any man's disciple—a grade most fit to rank beside the legendary *second* class of the nipponic Order of Chastity.

[3] *Mid-palmar space.*—A healthy, undissected man has no mid-palmar space—if " space " means " interval "; nor has he any popliteal space : *both* are convenient myths (though orthodox anatomists look coldly at Kanavel's). There is, however, in the hand between the palmar floor and ulnar bursa a fissile plane—an ' *espace décollable* ' that easily distends and shows a special shape when it becomes unstuck by pus or by injection.

carpal shaft, on the ulnar side of the volar face (Fig. 58). Between
these terminal attachments there is a small 'free' portion of
opponens belly, and this when isolated by a touch becomes the
palmar boundary of a loop-hole that is framed behind by fifth
metacarpal base and the joint it makes with unciform—the hamate
of B.N.A. (Fig. 58). An instrument thrust through this loop-hole

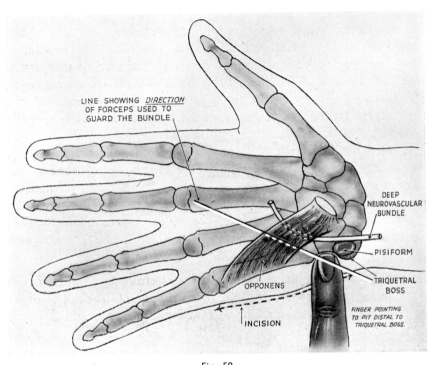

LINE SHOWING *DIRECTION*
OF FORCEPS USED TO
GUARD THE BUNDLE

DEEP
NEUROVASCULAR
BUNDLE

PISIFORM

OPPONENS

TRIQUETRAL
BOSS

*FINGER POINTING
TO PIT DISTAL TO
TRIQUETRAL BOSS.*

INCISION

Fig. 58

The landmarks

1. The triquetral boss from which the knife will cut along the edge of the fifth metacarpal.
2. The pit marked by the finger distal to the boss.   Opposite the pit we find the loop-hole
   to mid-palmar space.   A forceps *aimed* along the sloping line goes through the
   loop-hole *for a fingerbreadth* to form a tangent that will guard the curving ulnar bundle.

meets and overcomes a check; then it goes on and either penetrates mid-palmar space, or is a menace to the deep branch of
the ulnar nerve or to the ulnar bursa.

The hypothenar fascia.—The check is caused by the most radial
portion of a fascia that sheathes the hypothenar muscles and loops
them loosely, like a sling, to the shaft of fifth metacarpal. The
toughness of the membrane and its erratic spread to neighbouring
interosseous bellies vary in different persons.

The *deep branch of ulnar nerve* with its satellite artery and veins must be carefully avoided. The branch leaves the main trunk opposite the pisiform and sinks gradually into the palm between the two superficial muscles of the hypothenar group—abductor and short flexor of the little finger. It enters the field of operation as it grazes the ulnar side of the hamate (or unciform) hook and is there bridged or embraced by opponens fibres. Just distal to the hook the nerve and vessels fortunately bend thumb-wards, almost at right angles, and, fortunately again, the bend lies a good fingerbreadth radial to the loop-hole's mouth. Whatever instruments we turn toward the space will thus avoid the nerve if pointed distally—for choice, towards the *head* of third metacarpal (Fig. 58).

THE OPERATION

The site allows a long, benignly placed, incision, and this will give advantage for inspection combined with thorough drainage of a part where pus is liable to pocket. Blind use therefore of the loop-hole as a means of access should be condemned ; it is a mere lucky breach that must be *widened* for surgical attack.

Position.—With the patient recumbent under general anæs-thesia, either pronate and turn his upper limb till the *back* of the thumb rests on the table, or bring the half-pronated forearm into contact with the biceps. The first position has the merit of ulnar-flexing the hand and thus relaxing skin and muscle so that bony landmarks are easy to feel. At the moment, however, of making the incision the wrist should be propped straight to unwrinkle the skin.

Two ways of finding the pit which is the surface guide.—(1) Run a thumbnail down the ulnar border of the patient's *wrist* ; a thumb's breadth dorsal to the pisiform the nail will override a boss—the cuneiform or os triquetrum—and sink at once into a pit just distal to the boss. In this depression (which dips towards the loop-hole) the nail will touch the hard base of the fifth metacarpal immediately behind the hypothenar mass. (2) The thumb, slid proximally *up* the subcutaneous edge of fifth metacarpal, is checked by the triquetral boss exactly opposite the pit (Fig. 58).

The incision.—This begins on the triquetral boss and goes—through skin only—down the whole length of metacarpal edge ; skin and fat are reflected just sufficiently to show the bone and let us see the fascia that ensheathes the bulging belly of abductor—

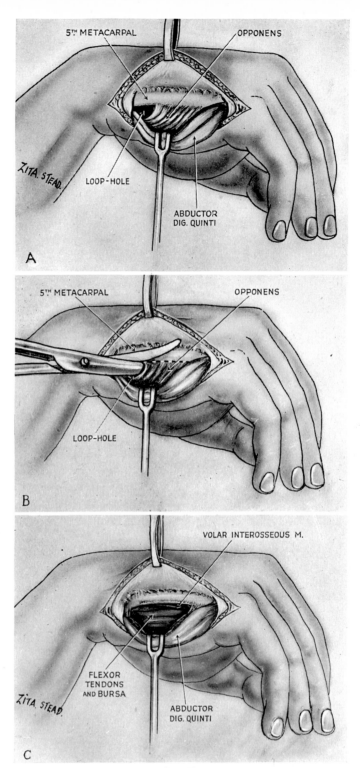

Fig. 59

The loop-hole and the exposure.—To find the loop-hole, A, slit the fascia binding abductor belly to the ulnar edge of fifth metacarpal. Retract the belly palmwards. Open a deeper fascia that lies just palmar to the metacarpal base. Deep to the fascia a touch of blunt dissection will dislodge the short 'free' portion of opponens towards the palm and so define the loop-hole. B. Widen the loop-hole by severing opponens. Open the fascia deep to the muscle. C. The ulnar bursa lies with its back to mid-palmar space.

a muscle recognised by its mobility before and during operation. Pick up this fascia close to the ulnar edge of metacarpal ; open it lengthwise without injuring abductor or the *dorsal* branch of ulnar nerve, which runs along the sheath ; liberate and retract the muscle palmwards. Then pick up and divide a thin fascia just in front of the metacarpal base.

It is now easy to define the loop-hole (Fig. 59) by raising the free portion of opponens from bone with the blunt nose of Mayo scissors ; withdraw and open the scissors ; pass one blade through the loop-hole and cut opponens close to metacarpal shaft, dividing all but distal fibres (Fig. 59) ; open the screen of fascia beyond. The ulnar bursa then appears—through the wide gap between hypothenar mass and palmar floor—bulging into the mid-palmar space (Fig. 59). Widen the gap still further by flexing the hand, especially its little finger. The deep neurovascular bundle can be protected during this operation with a closed forceps introduced along the palmar floor in the direction shown in Fig. 58—a safe-guard which I owe to Wing-Commander R. Shackman, my former colleague.

The final scar escapes the rubs of ordinary use.

MEDIAL APPROACH
TO THE DEEP TERMINAL BRANCH OF THE ULNAR NERVE

Exposures made through palmar skin can sometimes be exceedingly refractory ; and, if we use that route to deal with the deep ulnar branch, we split the palm from wrist to finger leaving the scar ill-placed.[1]

Instead we can adapt for this exposure the medial approach to the mid-palmar region (p. 77), prolonging the incision four fingerbreadths into the forearm (Fig. 61, A, below), disarticulating the pisiform, and—for the widest view—dividing the opponens.

THE OPERATION

After incising skin and fascia look for the ulnar trunk beside and radial to the tendon of flexor carpi ulnaris ; then trace it down to where it ends—just radial to pisiform—in deep and superficial branches. The *deep* branch lies next pisiform, and after trivial contact with its fellow nerve dips through the hypothenar mass.

[1] See Fig. 10 in a paper by C. A. Elsberg and A. H. Woods : *Archives of Neurology and Psychiatry*, 1919, **2**, 658.

We know already how to find the distal part of the deep branch
in the palm, opposite opponens loop-hole (p. 76) ; in order, therefore, to expose the nerve in continuity from the medial side we
must displace the interrupting block of pisiform.

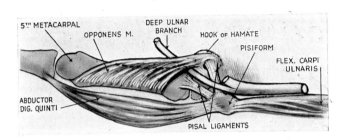

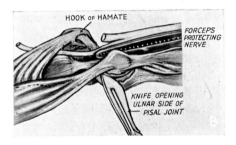

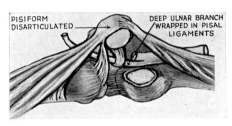

Fig. 60

Exposure of the deep terminal branch of ulnar nerve (anatomy)

Diagrams which show that when the pisiform is raised within its
band (like a patella), and turned in such a way that the articular
facet looks to the ulnar side, the pisal ligaments wrap round the
nerve. A. The undisturbed lay-out seen from its palmar aspect.
B and C are ulnar views : B. The pisal joint is opened while we
guard the nerve with intervening forceps ; C. The pisiform is raised
and turned to let the ligaments be cut in safety close to the facet.

Mobilising the pisiform.—The tendon of flexor carpi ulnaris
inserts on this bone, and abductor digiti quinti springs from it ; the
pisiform, therefore, detached from the wrist, remains (like a patella)
in the band formed by these muscles. The bone is also moored
by two ligaments which pass distally, and they are reinforced

with fibres from the tendon of flexor carpi ulnaris (Fig. 60) ; the weaker goes to the base of fifth metacarpal ; the other—a stout cord (crossed by the deep ulnar branch) goes to the hook of hamate. When therefore we lift the pisiform from its articulation (guarding the nerve with a metal tool while we divide the capsule of the joint) we see only the *start* of the branch ; the rest of its proximal portion is wrapped in ligaments (Fig. 60). These can be safely cut if the mobile bone (still in its band of muscle) is turned through a right angle so that the oval articular facet looks to the ulnar side ; then we divide the ligaments against the pisiform.

The deep branch may now be traced through fibres of abductor and opponens digiti quinti, and seen to great advantage (Fig. 61). But, if we need a wider access, dividing the opponens near the edge of metacarpal will let us reach two extra fingerbreadths of this short nerve (Fig. 61, c).

THE INNOCENT EFFECT OF PISAL DISARTICULATION

My readers should be warned. A piece of pure anatomy—most properly consigned in other pages of the book to footnotes—lies right ahead, and those who steadily pursue the by-pass of the text must now skip over an intrusion. But some that disarticulate the pisiform may wonder why they have not spoilt the ' flexor retina-culum ' (a recent alias of transverse carpal ligament). For in the current text-books which favour that nomenclature the proximal and ulnar corner of the retinaculum is fixed (they say) to pisiform. Detachment therefore of the pisiform should free the corner and impair restraint. It, happily, does nothing of the kind.

To think it might is to suppose that an important piece of band concerned in curbing tendons would be attached for *that* upon a mobile and unstable bone—an almost blasphemous conception.

Like every legend, this account of pisiform attachment is the distortion of a fact. There *is* a retinaculum whose proximal and ulnar corner is firmly fixed—not in a futile way to pisiform, but to the stable cuneiform (the os triquetrum of the Basle nomenclature). Then comes that old appurtenance of fairy-tale, the cloak of dark-ness : the cardinal attachment to the cuneiform is hidden under-neath extrinsic fibres from the pisal coat. These fibres spread in part from the insertion of flexor carpi ulnaris, and partly (on a deeper plane) from an oblique band that also coats the pisiform— a portion of the so-called *radio*carpal ligament. But far from working as a retinaculum this band (which springs, despite its

6

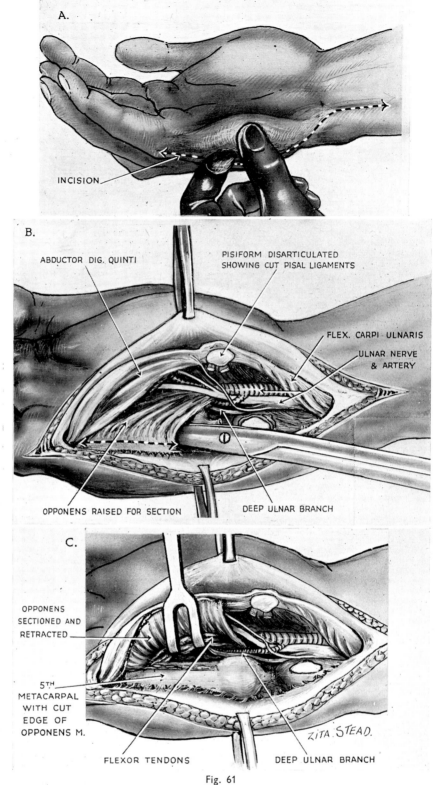

Fig. 61

Exposure of the deep ulnar branch (the operation)

A. Mobility test to find abductor digiti quinti ; incisions for the skin and fascia follow its dorsal edge and then go up the forearm—ulnar to flexor carpi tendon.

B. The disarticulated pisiform, detached from pisal ligaments, stays in its compound band. Obscuring fibres of opponens are cleared away to bare the nerve. For wider access mobilise opponens with Mayo scissors ; cut through the muscle close beside the edge of fifth metacarpal (B and C).

name, from ulnar styloid) *relaxes* when the wrist is palmar flexed. The retinaculum of course does not ; and it is just in virtue of its ulnar corner, fixed as it is to cuneiform, that flexor tendons are restrained from tearing pisiform away from carpus.

Current descriptions of this quondam transverse carpal ligament (once called anterior annular) call for revision. First, it is wrong, I think, to give the structure *as a whole* the name of flexor retinaculum ; it does not all by any means deserve it. Something also might be done to better the nomenclature which lumps as " radiocarpal " a ligamentous band whose proximal extremity springs only from the *ulna*—a band that may be found to play a part in wrenching off the styloid process in a Colles fracture.

The golden age of ligaments is gone. So has the silver age (with John Bland-Sutton) ; and rust begins to gather.

EXPOSURES IN THE LOWER LIMB

VESSELS AND NERVES IN THE BUTTOCK

I PUT this first. Of all exposures in the lower limb a method for the buttock was, I found, the principal concern of an experienced majority.

We have been taught to look for the gluteal vessels by splitting gluteus maximus, perhaps because its well-marked grain is almost irresistible. But if we split the grain, we play into the hands of entities that tend to give a narrow, bloody field. The parts are thick ; skin felts with fat, and fat with fascia covering thick gluteal muscle. Then, too, the vessels sprawl on the deep face of maximus, much as they sprawl on the placenta, spreading their arteries (as Bell remarks) " with sudden and crooked angles " ; so they diverge and run *across* the grain ; and here those cursed things of surgery, the veins, are large. These handicaps of mere anatomy grow uglier with wounds : the part becomes " a clotting mass adrip with blood."

In this exposure, therefore, we must spare and see—two things which can be done well only when we lift the lid-like shape of maximus as we might lift the lid nailed on a packing-case. Thus we can either raise the muscle by setting free a pair of sides that meet, and prising up the corner (like Fiolle and Delmas) ; or else (with Stookey)[1] we can set *two* corners free and turn the whole lid back. The plans themselves are simple, but neglect of detail leads to sorry execution.

ANATOMY

The gluteal lid.—(Fig. 62). The cover formed by maximus is like a parallelogram whose *shorter sides*—the femoral and pelvic— are almost longitudinal, the one aligning roughly with the femur, the other fixed from ilium to coccyx.

The *longer sides*—cephalic and caudal—are oblique, like the

---

[1] B. Stookey, *Journal of the American Medical Association*, 1920, **74**, 1380. (In the exposure described below, Stookey's ' question-mark ' has been shifted *forward* to exploit the Fiolle and Delmas drum-head.)

grain of maximus ; the lower side descends across the gluteal fold

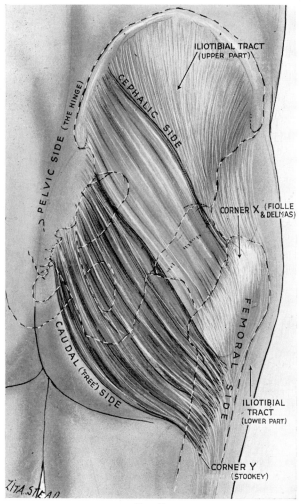

Fig. 62
The gluteal lid or parallelogram
Note its four sides—two long (cephalic and caudal), and two
short (femoral and pelvic). *All* the superficial fibres plus the
upper half of deep fibres are attached distally to iliotibial tract
(see Fig. 63). The lower (deeply shaded) half of the *deep*
fibres are fixed to femur. X is the corner to free in order to
prise up the lid in the partial exposure of Fiolle and Delmas.
Y is the second corner which must be freed with X to let us
raise the lid and hinge it back for the complete exposure, after
Stookey.

and is (as Boyer notes) the ' free ' side of the muscle—united to
surrounding parts by *loose* connective tissue.

Of these four sides two which meet in front—the short femoral, the long cephalic—need close consideration. All the fibres of gluteus maximus have their distal attachments at the short, *femoral side* of the muscle. These attachments are of two kinds, fascial and bony. The superficial fibres join the part of iliotibial tract which slides on great trochanter ; so, too, does the upper half of deeper fibres ; the lower half, however, implants itself on bone, marking the back of femur and forming there the distal point of the gluteal parallelogram.

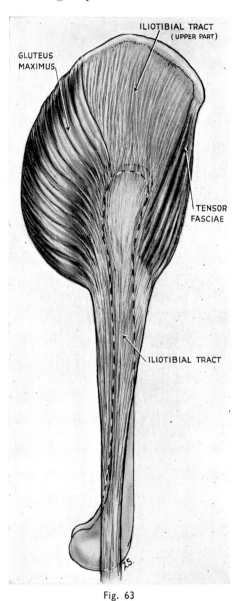

Fig. 63

The 'pelvic deltoid'

The fibrous middle part (formed by iliotibial tract) covers gluteus medius and is stuck to it in front. Behind, near great trochanter where medius slopes inward, the tract covers the muscle like a drum-head (see Fig. 66).

The long *cephalic side* that joins with the short femoral is bound, in muscle-sheath relation, to a special piece of tract—the proximal expanse which hides gluteus medius, and occupies the gap between the maximus and tensor muscle. Indeed, we may regard these three (the tensor, tract and maximus) as figuring a pelvic deltoid (Fig. 63) whose middle part consists of fibrous tissue—a useful myth in practice but one condemned by strict morphology.

If we set free these two adjoining sides—cephalic and femoral—dividing their attachments to the tract, we liberate a corner of gluteal lid which we can now prise up. But if we need the widest possible exposure (to reach in comfort, say, the great sciatic) we must unfix a second corner—

the distal piece of maximus that joins the femur. Then every side is free except the pelvic; for (as we know from Boyer) the caudal edge is virtually unattached. And so, with three sides free, we raise the lid.

THE OPERATIONS OF PARTIAL AND COMPLETE EXPOSURE

Position.—The patient lies face down. Take advantage of this position to mark out the points through which the knife will pass : (1) the posterior superior spine of ilium ; (2) a point on the crest a handbreadth in front of this ; (3) most difficult of all to find, a point midway between the front edge and the back edge of great trochanter. (Be sure you find the front *edge* under the covering wad of tensor belly) ; (4) a similar point on the femoral shaft level with gluteal fold ; (5) a point on the back of thigh midway between ischial tuberosity and the back of great trochanter, just below the gluteal fold (Fig. 64).

The skin incision.—Since it is difficult to know beforehand if our exposure must be full or partial, I shall describe the full incision—a question-mark on the right side, its mirror image on the left (Fig. 64)—and indicate the portion that gives room for *circumscribed* approach.

The ' question-mark ' needs rigorous attention ; a lapse will hamper us persistently.[1] Begin first at the posterior superior spine of ilium ; carry the knife a handbreadth along the iliac crest. Then cut obliquely down the outer face of hip to reach the top of great trochanter. The knife proceeding distally bisects the outer face of the trochanter and travels down the shaft till level with the gluteal fold ; *that* is enough for circumscribed exposure. But, for full access turn the knife in transversely at this level ; stop at the midline of the thigh, half-way, that is, between the great trochanter and the tuberosity of ischium. Then cut vertically down the thigh as far as you propose to liberate the great sciatic nerve. The ' question-mark ' should reach but not divide deep fascia.

The posterior cutaneous nerve of the thigh.—The *trunk* of this large nerve (once named the small sciatic) lies in the midline of the thigh just under the deep fascia ; *and there it stays*, sending out perforating twigs and coming to the surface only in the calf

---

[1] It is, for example, remarkably (and ruinously) easy to follow the hinder edge of great trochanter instead of bisecting its outer face—

> " *I told them once, I told them twice :*
> *They would not listen to advice.*"

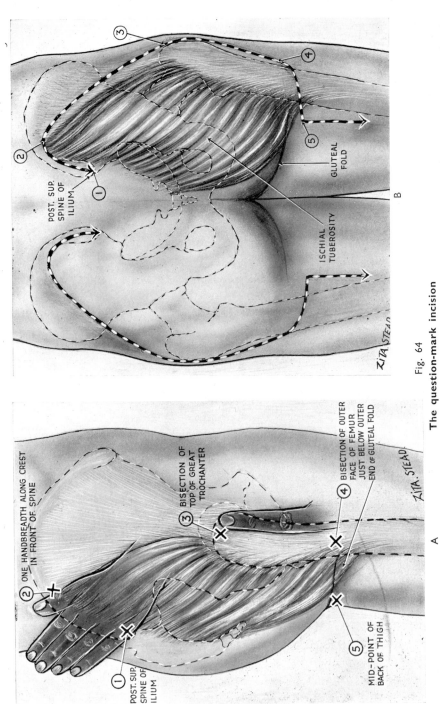

Fig. 64

The question-mark incision

A. Note the five points which map its course. The 'difficult' point (3) is a fingerbreadth behind the front edge of great trochanter. For the partial exposure of Fiolle and Delmas, incision stops at point 4. B shows the full 'question-mark' on the right; its mirror image on the left.

Labels in figure B:
- ③
- ④
- ②
- ⑤
- ①
- POST. SUP. SPINE OF ILIUM
- GLUTEAL FOLD
- ISCHIAL TUBEROSITY
- B
- ZITA STEAD

Labels in figure A:
- ② ONE HANDBREADTH ALONG CREST IN FRONT OF SPINE
- ③ BISECTION OF TOP OF GREAT TROCHANTER
- ④ BISECTION OF OUTER FACE OF FEMUR JUST BELOW OUTER END OF GLUTEAL FOLD
- ① POST. SUP. SPINE OF ILIUM
- ⑤ MID-POINT OF BACK OF THIGH
- A
- ZITA STEAD

(Fig. 65). This nerve will be imperilled by a full exposure; it clings, ensheathed in fat, to the deep face of maximus, close to the long ' free ' caudal edge. So, when the edge is raised, the nerve is cut unless we make a point of finding it *as a first step*, using the *stem* of the ' question-mark ' — a method which I owe to Major C. W. Clark of the Canadian Army. His plan works well, for nerve and stem are mesially placed. The nerve, remember, lies beneath deep fascia (and just beneath); so we can find it much more easily than if it lay in superficial fat. Open deep fascia therefore longitudinally and trace the trunk up to the edge of the gluteal lid. When presently we raise the lid and hinge it back, the nerve is easily detached—together with its perineal branch, the *ci-devant* pudendal nerve of Sœmmerring.

Liberation of the adjoining femoral and cephalic sides.—We next set free the shorter, *femoral* side of maximus by cutting down on bone and splitting lengthwise the piece of iliotibial tract that slides on shaft and great trochanter. Our cut accordingly bisects the outer surface of the femur and divides the main (and fascial) insertion of the maximus (Figs. 64, A and 65).

We then proceed to free the long, *cephalic* side of maximus, which, as we know already, is fastened by a sheet of iliotibial tract; and this we must divide. A detail of arrangement makes it well to place the cut correctly.

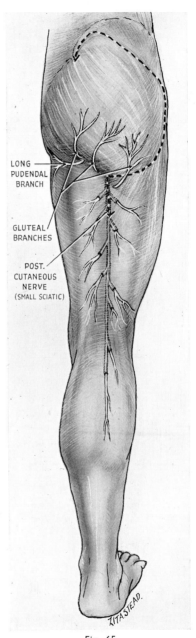

LONG PUDENDAL BRANCH

GLUTEAL BRANCHES

POST. CUTANEOUS NERVE (SMALL SCIATIC)

Fig. 65

The posterior cutaneous nerve of the thigh (the small sciatic)

Note its long course under deep fascia. Find it through the *stem* of the ' question-mark,' and thus, with C. W. Clark, protect the nerve (which sticks to the deep face of maximus)*before* you mobilise the caudal edge of the gluteal lid.

The useful drum-head.—This sheet of tract (the fibrous portion of the pelvic ' deltoid ') covers the several parts of gluteus medius with different degrees of contiguity. In front, the tract and muscle stick together ; behind, the two are separate. So, when medius is lax, it leaves the hinder piece of tract stretched like a drum-head over it. The opening of this drum-head through a small extension upwards of the cut already made along the femur will let us put a finger in the shallow cavity and use a thumb to grasp the rubbery

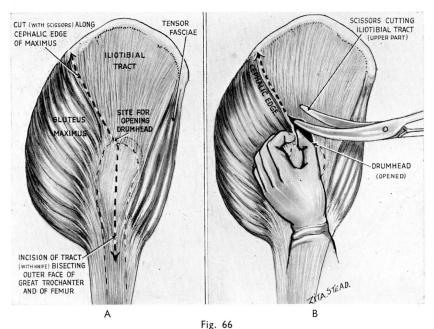

A   B

Fig. 66

Line for dividing iliotibial tract

A. The *knife* bisects the outer face of great trochanter and of femur ; it opens the drum-head at the top of the bisection. B. Finger and thumb locate the rubbery cephalic edge of maximus, and *scissors* cut the tract along beside it. Knife and scissors thus detach the *first* corner of the lid (X in Fig. 62) by setting free its femoral and cephalic sides.

transition that marks the meeting-place of maximus and tract. Use scissors to divide the tract along this sloping edge (Fig. 66).

And now with two sides free we raise one corner of the lid and look for structures underneath. That is the method of Fiolle and Delmas. But for fuller view we must set free a second corner.

The second corner of the lid.—We have already found the ' free,' or caudal, edge of maximus along with the posterior cutaneous nerve (once called the small sciatic). Raise both together from the hamstrings. Hook a finger round and then cut through the

thick insertion of maximus to femur ; the muscle there is sometimes vascular and should be pressed between assistant fingers on
the medial side of the dividing knife (Fig. 67).   Before we turn

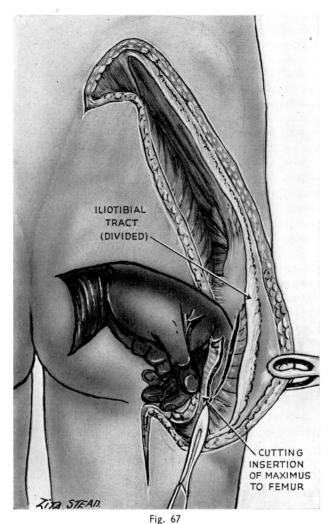

ILIOTIBIAL
TRACT
(DIVIDED)

CUTTING
INSERTION
OF MAXIMUS
TO FEMUR

ZITA STEAD.

Fig. 67
Freeing the second corner (Y in Fig. 62)
This is done by dividing the fleshy attachment of maximus to femur.
Fingers control the proximal extremity which is often vascular.

the muscle over we must see that the posterior cutaneous nerve is
finally detached and safe. The whole gluteal lid can then be hinged
back on its pelvic fastening, but very gently ; for though the great
arterial and venous stems that branch into the lid are favourably
placed—close to the pelvic hinge—the veins are always weak, and,
in the old, the arteries are brittle.

STRUCTURES UNDER THE GLUTEAL LID

The key and the trap.—There is a key muscle for this region ; each main nerve and vessel leaves the pelvis at one or other edge of pyriformis ; and as a rule we find this ' key ' immediately. Sometimes, however, a deep fold in gluteus medius marks off a neighbouring piece of belly close beside the ' key ' (Fig. 68) ; then a small effort will separate the hinder part of medius into a disconcerting replica of pyriformis. I have twice seen confusion follow this detachment. (The transverse plane grazing the top of great trochanter is at the caudal edge of pyriformis—a muscle sometimes fused above with medius and minimus.)

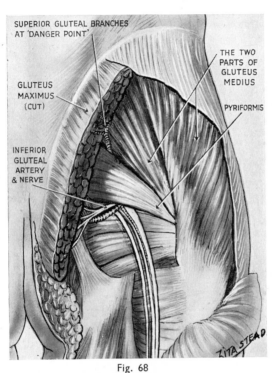

SUPERIOR GLUTEAL BRANCHES AT 'DANGER POINT'

THE TWO PARTS OF GLUTEUS MEDIUS

GLUTEUS MAXIMUS (CUT)

PYRIFORMIS

INFERIOR GLUTEAL ARTERY & NERVE

Fig. 68

Pitfalls under the gluteal lid

Note the posterior part of gluteus medius which is sometimes separated off and mistaken for pyriformis, causing complete disorientation. Note also the ' danger spot ' where a branch of superior gluteal artery, accompanied by *veins*, spreads into maximus. It lies three fingerbreadths in front of the posterior superior spine of ilium and three fingerbreadths below the crest.

The muscles.— Seven *transverse* muscular parts cross the wound from above down: the hinder piece of gluteus medius, pyriformis, gemellus superior, the tendon of obturator internus, gemellus inferior, quadratus femoris, adductor magnus. The *vertical* muscles seen under the lid are proximal parts of the hamstrings (Fig. 69). A narrow tongue, more deeply placed, and lateral to where the fleshy fibres of maximus insert on femur, is vastus lateralis.

Structures related to the borders of pyriformis.—At its *upper edge* are the superior gluteal vessels and nerve. The nerve runs forward with offsets of the vessels, and is concealed at once by gluteus medius. The artery and *large* companion veins continue

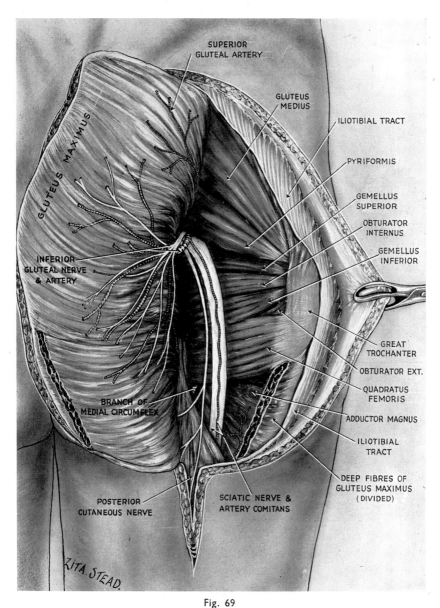

Fig. 69

The gluteal lid hinged back

The exposure is completed except in respect of the subgluteal arc formed by pudendal bundle (see the next figure—Fig. 70). Biceps is left in place to stress the fact that on its way to fibula the sloping belly crosses the sciatic. Therefore in following the nerve prolong the stem of 'question-mark' and mobilise the biceps : raise the belly like a bucket-handle and trace the nerve deep to it. (Only the *infrabicipital* part of sciatic lies between inner and outer hamstrings.)

into maximus and constitute a veritable danger spot—three finger-breadths in front of the posterior superior spine of ilium and three below the crest—a point to keep in mind when hinging back the lid.

At the *lower edge of pyriformis* the most superficial structure to emerge is the inferior gluteal nerve whose trunk breaks up at once in branches of supply to maximus and screens the lower gluteal vessels. These last send offsets down beside the structure next in depth—the small sciatic or posterior cutaneous nerve, already seen and spared (p. 89). It lay (before we had displaced it) along the posteromedial edge of the " huge great sciatic nerve "—the one oasis of description Gogarty could find in ' Cunningham '[1] (Figs. 68 and 69).

Still deeper is the nerve to quadratus femoris—deep to the gemelli group and reaching the *deep* face of its own muscle. Its course is covered by a finger laid beside and lateral to the ischial tuberosity.

The internal pudendal bundle.—This, too, emerges at the lower edge of pyriformis, curving between the great and small sciatic notch, and lying deep and slightly medial to the lower gluteal screen of nerves and vessels—a source of hæmorrhage to think of once gluteals are controlled, and one whereon we might be called to pounce ; which we can do as follows.

FINDING THE SITE OF THE PUDENDAL BUNDLE.—Use the left hand for the right side, and *vice versa*. Abduct the thumb *widely*. Slide the forefinger up across the sciatic trunk and then along the back of the ischial tuberosity. Keep the palmar surface of the finger flat against the bone and let the distal phalanx pass deep to pyriformis, into the great sciatic notch. The finger will advance until the web of the outstretched thumb is stopped against the great trochanter (Fig. 70). Then the tip of the finger, slightly flexed, will press on the arc of the pudendal bundle ; this as a rule sticks fast to its background and will not let itself be hooked without a little blunt dissection.[2]

Thus, after hinging back the gluteal lid, a single rapid movement finds the bundle and allows precise insertion of a tampon (Mikulicz for choice). This may stop the bleeding, or, at least,

---

[1] Failure to realise that the long head of biceps slopes across the back of sciatic may cause confusion—especially if we attempt to trace the nerve through insufficient stems of ' question-marks ' (see Fig. 69, and legend).

[2] The bundle, one should know, consists of three parts : pudendal vessels flanked by two nerves. The vessels lie more or less on the tip of the ischial spine ; the internal pudendal nerve is on the inner side of the vessels; the small nerve to obturator internus (which also gives a twig to gemellus superior) lies on their outer side.

will stanch it and give time to reach and tie the parent trunk by means of laparotomy.

Repair.—We must most carefully reconstitute the field of operation—especially the proximal expanse of iliotibial tract.

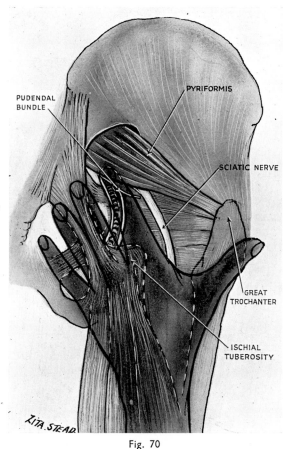

Fig. 70

Finding the pudendal bundle

Using the left hand for the right side and vice versa, the index slides on the tendon-covered back of ischial tuberosity, lengthwise, till the hand is stopped by great trochanter making contact with the web of the outstretched thumb. The tip of index passes *deep* to pyriformis into the great sciatic notch and comes to rest on the pudendal bundle.

Smooth function here depends on normal interplay of all three portions of the pelvic ' deltoid '—of tensor, tract and maximus. A hernial defect (with bulging of gluteus medius) may lead to snapping-hip, or to recurring, noiseless subluxation of tract on great trochanter. In either case the consequent imbalance makes and unmakes a postural deformity which certain temperaments are haunted by, and some (however innocent) exploit.[1]

THE ROLE OF GLUTEUS MAXIMUS IN CERTAIN MOVEMENTS

A sitting man cannot raise himself if the part of his body which is in front of his centre of gravity does not weigh more than that which is behind his centre of gravity without the use of his arms.

The sinew which guides the leg, and which is connected with the patella of the knee, feels it a greater labour to carry the man upwards in proportion as the knee is more bent ; and the muscle which acts upon the angle made by the thigh where it joins the body has less difficulty and has less weight to lift because it has not the additional weight of the thigh itself. And besides it has the stronger muscles, being those which form the buttock.[2]   LEONARDO DA VINCI.

If when you grasp a muscle you can shift it easily from side to side, you may be sure the muscle is relaxed sufficiently to make it—at the moment of your test—unfit to work as a prime mover. That state of idle relaxation is the state of maximus in most of the activities which text-books claim for it [3] (though fingers must be careful not to take for its contraction the *neighbouring* activity of hamstrings).

[1] Two examples : (1) Gluteus medius hernia (after Ober's operation of fascial division for backache) which caused undue preoccupation with shifting aspects of a great trochanter. (2) A rather simple individual with snapping hip, who drew a useful pension for " recurring *dislocation* " of the joint. A loud click synchronised with three-inch shortening of the limb—apparent, but extremely lucrative.

[2] These are in no way final and decisive statements : each is a *note*—" the shadow of a thought in process of formation."

[3] A pair of these accounts (with comments in parenthesis) appear below. They may, I think, be handled as unfeelingly as fossilised remains : the uncoordinated " actions " of a single muscle are parentless survivals, out of date since the Renaissance.

   From Gray's Anatomy, 1942, 28*th Edn., p.* 634.—" When the Gluteus maximus takes its fixed point from the pelvis, it extends the thigh and brings it into line with the trunk." [*The muscle is lax during the movement.*] " Taking its fixed point below, it supports the pelvis and the trunk upon the head of the femur, and, so far as the hip-joint is concerned, the maintenance of the erect attitude is ensured by the balanced tone of the Gluteus maximus and the other extensors of the joint, on the one hand, and of the flexors of the joint on the other hand." [*The maximus is absolutely lax in static natural erect positions, but if we spring to full ' attention ', and (in our zeal) incline to thrust the pelvis forward, it thrusts the pelvis forward* (see footnote p. 98),—*a fault that has no part in keeping us erect.*] " Its most powerful action is to raise the trunk after stooping by drawing the pelvis backward." [*The maximus is lax throughout the movement.*] " It is a tensor of the fascia lata, and through the iliotibial tract it steadies the femur on the tibia during standing when the extensor muscles are relaxed." [*See the last comment but one, above.*]

   From Cunningham's Text-Book of Anatomy, 1943, 8*th Edn., p.* 508.—" The gluteus maximus is mainly an extensor of the thigh and has a powerful action in straightening the

The muscle, for example, is relaxed if we extend the hip ; in standing still ; in rising from the exercise of touching toes with straightened knees ; in leaning back when seated. Tradition has enjoined on maximus the task of moving *back* the femur and the pelvis. These movements in reverse are fortunately absent, else we should never climb the stairs, or leave a seat by voluntary act : gluteus maximus would guarantee that we were damned (like Sisyphus) to lasting retropulsion.

The muscle works quite otherwise. Taking a fixed and distal point in front, at the insertion of the ilio*tibial* tract upon the *front* of the tibia, its action (leaving seats or mounting stairs) helps to effect the raising of the pelvis and the femur *forward*, strapping each to each in such a way as to combine great solidarity with requisite mobility.[1]

The task indeed seems herculean, befitting well the bulk of maximus. But looking closer at the muscle we find the *length* of fibre far too short for the achievement : it measures roughly half the length of the required range of movement, and even maximal contraction could only bring the trunk through less than quarter of the path it actually travels to surmount the foot.

I think it therefore possible that maximus may work instead like a *supporting* giant—a kind of Atlas—bearing the body's weight on fleshy hands while quadriceps, relieved of strain, procures the movement up and forward of a mass maintained at every stage in levitation.

What happens when, unaided by our arms, we rise to full

---

lower limb, as in climbing or running." [*Does this imply : when acting from its origin ? For presently we find the phrase :* " Acting from its insertion "—*as if to signify antithesis. If the antithesis is meant, the words suggest a retropulsion during climbing, just as they did when used in* 1922 (5th Edn., p. 417).] " Its lower fibres also adduct the thigh and rotate it laterally." [*The fibres meanwhile are relaxed.*] " Acting from its insertion the muscle is a powerful extensor of the trunk when the body is being raised from the sitting or stooping position ; " [*But these are movements made in* opposite *directions : the trunk moves forward from the sitting posture ; backward from the stooping posture.*]

Perhaps, since 1498, sufficient time has passed to let our text-books try the plan of Leonardo and link the muscles with descriptions of our common *acts*. Their total is, he notes, eighteen—a figure whose correction would do nothing to reduce his genius or evince a trace of it in others.

[1] The *femur* is slung forward as a whole by maximus in virtue of the junction which the lateral intermuscular septum makes with the part of iliotibial tract that constitutes the tendon of maximus. The septum at its inner edge is fixed to linea aspera ; its outer edge, as we shall see below (p. 120 and Fig. 87, B), joins with the hinder border of the tract. And so, by way of tract and septum, maximus secures a purchase on the shaft throughout its length.

The ' strap ' effect is due to *tightening* of the tract whose pressure on the great trochanter forces the backward-sloping neck to drive and hold the head of femur up against the *front* of acetabulum.

height from a chair ?   Before we leave the seat the trunk tilts
slightly towards the knees—a movement due, I think, to iliopsoas,
not to rectus femoris. The feet are usually drawn back, and thus
reduce the distance which the trunk must go to reach a stable
equilibrium. Then both the maximi contract, and—like a pair of
hands passed from in front to curve behind the pelvis—begin to
lift the trunk and thigh (this last through the iliotibial tract and
lateral septum, see p. 120) together forward on the legs. In front the
quadriceps conducts the movement. And then surprisingly, while
hip and knee are still in flexion, first maximi, then recti, cease to
act and leave the *final* straightening of the limb to semitendinosus.[1]

This action of a hamstring may seem strange, because we learn
(by rote) to call the hamstrings "*flexors* of the knee." And so
they are—provided that the foot is off the ground and quadriceps
is lax. But the semitendinosus differs from its fellow hamstrings :
it is attached in front of—not behind—the ' centre ' for the movement of the knee ; its lower tendon curves like fingers round the
lever of the tibial shaft. So, when the foot is standing firm, and
while the ankle acts as fulcrum, then a contraction of the muscle
will pull the top of the tibia *back* and bring the knee to full
extension. And you will find that if the trunk is vertical (and
therefore does not need the aid of other hamstrings to check
a forward plunge), semitendinosus, alone of all the local bellies
you can feel, is genuinely taut throughout the movement.   It is,
in fact, a service-pattern ' muscle of attention '.

A model made in plasticine of the half pelvis seems to throw
further light. Let it be flat at first, on the Mercator principle ;
string it with thread attached like maximus from ilium to coccyx
and thence continued into ' iliotibial tract '. Pivot the slab upon
its ' acetabulum ' ; pull the loop forwards, letting your hand sink

---

[1] The sudden laxity of maximus is fortunate perhaps if we consider how the *hyper*active
muscle lifts the pelvis nearly to the summit of the arch of opisthotonus produced by
strychnine or by tetanus, in gross exaggeration of the movement which a patient makes
to let the nurse remove a bed-pan. In this routine event the quadriceps is not protagonist,
and maximus, behaving now as a *protrusor of the pelvis*, must put forth all its strength—
a thing it rarely does, leaving to other muscles acts it might perform, and working when
it must ; and then with notable economies of effort.

That is a common character of muscle. A palmar flexion of my wrist against the
force of gravity, and made with fingers loose, tightens the tendon of my flexor carpi
radialis, which stands out like a ridge. Then, if I close my grip, the radialis ridge goes
limp and fades, throwing the work instead upon a broader ridge of finger flexors. A
loosening of the grip restores the *status quo* : the radialis juts ; the finger tendons fade.
And while the order of this devolution fluctuates in wrists which (unlike mine) possess
a long-palmaris tendon, the principle remains. No wonder, therefore, that we sometimes
note a will to do the minimum and ' pass the buck ' ; these traits—united with the
most unhuman *readiness*—are in the grain of all our striped activity.

slowly as it pulls. Almost at once the ' semi-pelvis ' tilts. Now mould the plasticine which stands for ilium in close accordance with the bone : make it look backward at its hinder part, and splay it out ; stagger the ' coccyx ' inward from the ' ischium '. Pulling once more you find that a large fraction of the force which made the model nod when it was flat is now absorbed in twisting it : the downward pull instead of causing an immediate nutation begins to turn the slab in such a way that if the plasticine were living bone the pubis would be forced towards its fellow at the symphysis, and ilium would try to wrench itself away from sacrum.

Here—in connection with nutation—our plasticine perhaps illuminates the problem of the deeper caudal piece of maximus affixed to the gluteal mark : the fibres ought, one feels, to pull the upper part of femur *back*. Yet, if we force the thigh to full extension on the trunk, and then as far as it will go behind the buttock, though hamstrings harden, maximus is limp. And, when we rise from chairs, the upper part of femur travels *forward*. (The only backward-moving portion is the lower end—drawn backwards as we saw (p. 98), by semitendinosus when maximus had *ceased* to act.) Possibly these caudal fibres help in countering the forward inclination of the pelvis produced by rectus femoris and upper parts of maximus.

With plasticine (as in the art of surgery) experience may be fallacious ; but, as one handles it, a feeling grows that maximus could play a Titan's part—moulding the shape of pelvis, and redoubling special portions of the bone predestined to *withstand* the stress of moulding—a dual part that might be found to mark, for anthropologists the hillman, say, from certain dwellers on the plain. And, if the skull shape alters rapidly with new environment (as Ridgeway thought in 1908, and Boas tried to prove in 1912),[1] may not the shape of pelvis too ? Or could a faster change, in favour this time of obstetrics, be got by early training of the muscle ?

It seems, perhaps, that Aristophanes was right when (in the *Clouds*) he let his students of astronomy look skyward with their rumps : gluteal muscles bring a host of problems into focus.

---

[1] Sir W. Ridgeway, 1908, *Presidential Address to the Section of Anthropology*, British Association for the Advancement of Science ; Franz Boas, 1912, *Changes in Bodily Form of Descendants of Immigrants*, Washington D.C. 61st Congress, 2nd Session, State Documents 64, Document No. 208.

The care of convalescent maximi.—A brace of simple rules emerge from these conceptions. The patient, while recumbent, must be *lifted* on to bed-pans in order to prevent the all-out effort of the maximus that goes with a protrusion of the pelvis (see footnote, p. 98). Then, when he leaves the bed, we *lift* him to his feet and keep him on the level. There he may walk (gently and making short steps) with maximi as limp as battle-dress—a gait that we must teach *before* the patients rise. (In normal gait the fibres of the maximus stretch while the moving limb swings past its fellow, till, as we ground the heel, they harden suddenly—a little on the flat, but more and more with rise of gradient. Contracting thus they help the pelvis on to overtake the foot.)

So, in his *early* convalescence, the patient need not use the damaged maximus ; and if, as well, we lower him to sit or lie and do not let him stoop, he will not strain its fibre.

THE FRONT OF FEMUR

This (like its brachial homologue) is covered by a half-sleeve of muscle ; and whether we explore the back of humerus or front of femur our practice is identical : we look first for a *seam*, then open it to find a deep head coating bone and crossed obliquely by a neurovascular bundle. Accordingly to reach the shaft in either case we rip the seam, loop the bundle and split the deep head.

I shall return to these points later.

APPROACH TO THE FEMORAL SHAFT FROM IN FRONT

Exposure of the femur from the outer side was once the fashion : it called for no reflection—the surgeon cut directly down on bone. The inconvenient, unsightly and bloody wound seemed to suggest a price exacted for security, together with a certain disregard of structure. The knife thus used transects the slanting fibres of vastus lateralis, a goal of all four perforating arteries and of the branch descending from the outer circumflex. The patient, too, must lie upon his side, or else the surgeon works at disadvantage.

The method found below[1] respects anatomy, is relatively blood-less, and gives a wide exposure : over twelve inches of the *shaft—*

---

[1] *British Journal of Surgery*, 1924, **12**, 84.

from small trochanter to the lower end—are easily accessible. We look in comfort on the front and sides of femur; and while the patient still lies flat, we can secure a safe, dependent drainage.

Let us now take up the points of the first paragraph.

The *half-sleeve* consists of the quadriceps, enclosed in fascia; its seam (which shapes the course of our incision) lies between vastus lateralis and rectus femoris—a pair of heads that part towards their origins and form a V-shaped entrance to the sleeve. This entrance will be found a handbreadth distal to the great trochanter, in line, of course, with the incision which runs from anterior superior spine down to the outer angle of patella (Figs. 71 and 72). For further guidance grasp the long and relatively mobile rectus head below the 'spine', and move the muscle crosswise; the outer margin of the mobile zone will mark the seam.

The upper part of Fig. 71 shows that we must separate two other bellies—sartorius and tensor fasciæ—a very simple act for those who take the care to mark out incisions precisely. Then when the seam is ripped two structures must be kept in mind before exposing bone—suprapatellar pouch and neurovascular bundle.

The neurovascular bundle.—Coating the femur, when we rip the sleeve, we see a silvery fish-like belly—the deep, investing belly of crureus (or vastus intermedius in B.N.A.). A bundle slopes across its face consisting of the nerve (or nerves) to vastus lateralis plus outer branches (with companion veins) of lateral circumflex artery. This bundle can be found—in providential fat—a handbreadth distal to the great trochanter; and when it has been mobilised and looped up like a bucket-handle, *then* we can split the muscle deep to it and reach the shaft (Fig. 74).

The *suprapatellar pouch* spreads, when the limb is straight, three fingerbreadths above patella. Pouch and bundle are described below in further detail.

THE OPERATION

Position.—With the patient flat on his back, extend the knee on the side of operation; then raise the heel well off the table, relaxing rectus femoris.

Incision.—Divide the skin (and afterwards deep fascia) from anterior superior iliac spine to the outer angle of patella (Fig. 71). It is important to make this cut in such a way that we can open fascia *between* the tensor muscle and sartorius.

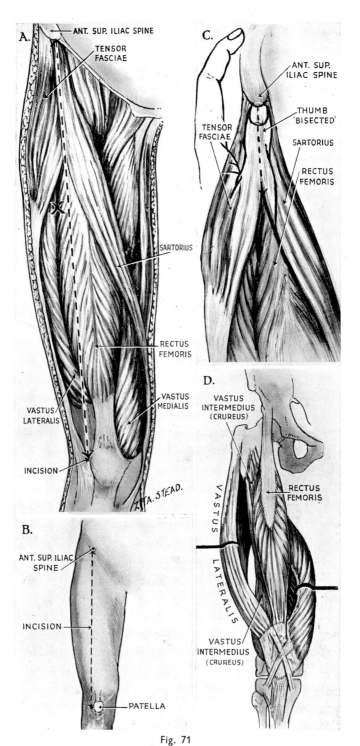

Fig. 71

The quadriceps sleeve in relation to the anterior incision

The cut goes from anterior superior spine to the outer angle of patella—close to the seam between rectus femoris ant outer vastus (A and B). Find the entrance, X, to the sleeve one handbreadth below the top of great trochanter (or *two* handbreadths below anterior superior spine). From there the seam rips easily. The common mistake is to make the cut too far out. Avoid this by catching the thumb-nail squarely under the *notch* of the ' spine ' (C). The knife ' bisects ' the thumb and parts sartorius from tensor fasciæ. D (*after* Poirier) shows the segments of the sleeve, and how part of vastus intermedius (crureus) lies *behind* the distal half of vastus lateralis.

Begin exactly at the centre of the very shallow notch immediately below the spine.

It is impossible to find it by approaching from above; feel therefore from below. The thumb does this best, catching the notch with its nail. A cut can then be made as if to split the thumb

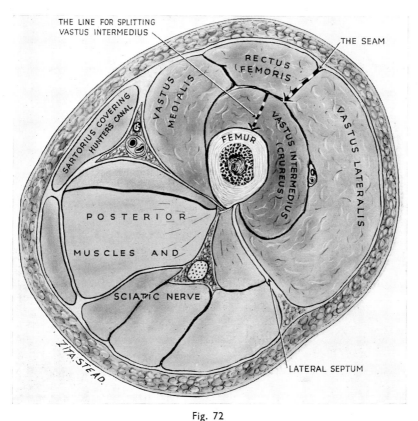

Fig. 72

The quadriceps sleeve in cross-section

Note the position of the seam, which must be ripped, and the line for splitting vastus intermedius—the deep, investing head which coats the femur.

in half (Fig. 71). The common error is to choose too lateral a point; the knife strays into muscle and butchery begins.

Planes of cleavage.—The finger finds the V-like interval between rectus femoris and vastus lateralis, a handbreadth distal to the great trochanter; and passing down between the bellies meets with minor vessels, which are caught and cut. More distally the finger will be checked where the vastus fibres join the rectus margin; then we use a knife.

The trilaminar tendon of quadriceps.—A working knowledge here will let us rip the sleeve still farther down and thus obtain a maximal exposure.

The stout component from the rectus femoris lies in a groove provided by the distal parts of medial and lateral vasti (Fig. 73). Adjacent portions of these vasti, flush with rectus tendon, fasten on its borders and send their deeper fibres of insertion round behind to make a common sheet which cradles it. This interwoven sheet (the second lamina) lies on the third and deepest—formed, of course, by tendon from the vastus intermedius (the part of quadriceps once called crureus).

So, if we wish to mobilise the distal portion of the rectus and

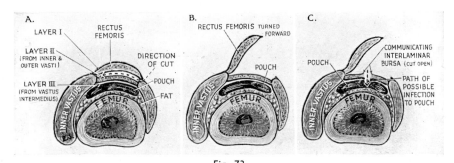

Fig. 73

Delamination and rotation of quadriceps tendon to secure further distal exposure of shaft

A. Divide the edge of rectus tendon from vastus lateralis ; then, with the knife laid flat, detach the *back* of rectus tendon down to patella. This will let you twist the tendon (B)— and, with it, all the rectus—farther forward, exposing more of vastus intermedius *belly*. (In order to avoid the pouch, the splitting of intermedius belly (Fig. 74) is checked four finger-breadths above patella—a point which lies, of course, above the level shown in these pictures.) Note the fat between pouch and bone, which (with the extra access got by delamination) lets us separate the pouch intact and reach the distal limit of the shaft. C. Shows the theoretical risk of delamination in presence of sepsis—if any interlaminar bursa should happen to communicate with suprapatellar pouch.

bare the shaft still farther down, we separate at first the *edge* of rectus tendon from the vastus lateralis ; then, with the knife blade in the frontal plane, we cleave its hinder surface from the vastus sheet and so delaminate the tendon of the quadriceps (Fig. 73). After this cleavage we can twist the outer edge of rectus *as a whole* much farther forward and so get extra room to see and split the fish-like, bone-investing belly of the vastus intermedius.

The frontal cut to cleave the laminæ of quadriceps should not be made in presence of infection : bursæ are found at times between the layers, and might (if they were sliced, and chanced as well to join with the synovial pouch) bring sepsis to the knee (Fig. 73, c).

The neurovascular bundle.—Now that the sleeve is ripped the slanting bundle shows, a handbreadth distal to the top of great

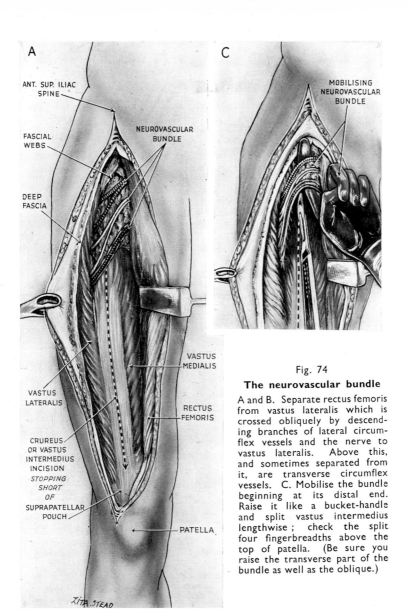

A

ANT. SUP. ILIAC SPINE

FASCIAL WEBS

NEUROVASCULAR BUNDLE

DEEP FASCIA

VASTUS MEDIALIS

VASTUS LATERALIS

RECTUS FEMORIS

CRUREUS OR VASTUS INTERMEDIUS INCISION *STOPPING SHORT OF* SUPRAPATELLAR POUCH

PATELLA

ZITA STEAD

C

MOBILISING NEUROVASCULAR BUNDLE

Fig. 74

The neurovascular bundle

A and B. Separate rectus femoris from vastus lateralis which is crossed obliquely by descending branches of lateral circumflex vessels and the nerve to vastus lateralis. Above this, and sometimes separated from it, are transverse circumflex vessels. C. Mobilise the bundle beginning at its distal end. Raise it like a bucket-handle and split vastus intermedius lengthwise ; check the split four fingerbreadths above the top of patella. (Be sure you raise the transverse part of the bundle as well as the oblique.)

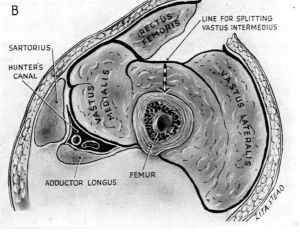

B

SARTORIUS

HUNTER'S CANAL

RECTUS FEMORIS

LINE FOR SPLITTING VASTUS INTERMEDIUS

VASTUS MEDIALIS

VASTUS LATERALIS

ADDUCTOR LONGUS

FEMUR

ZITA STEAD

trochanter. The nerves and vessels reach the outer vastus and sink into it. Often they spread out fanwise (as in Fig. 74) or else divide into quadrants, two or three in number. A thin transparent fascia binds them (with surrounding streaks of fat) to vastus intermedius. The presence of this fat makes mobilising easy. Division of the binding film along the lowest streak will often let us raise the bundle as a whole upon the finger— like a bucket-handle. An upper transverse part is sometimes missed through carelessness; and sometimes quadrants widely separate may need a further opening of the film.

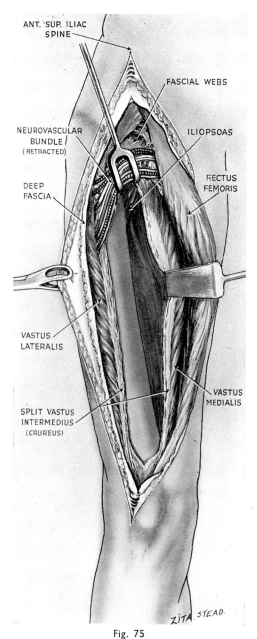

Fig. 75

Anterior exposure of femur

Detach the split vastus intermedius and expose as much of the shaft as you wish.

Under this arching 'handle' cut to bone by splitting through the length of vastus intermedius. Watch for sharp bleeding from a vein divided in the upper fibres.

The suprapatellar pouch. —Avoid a penetration of this pouch which spreads three fingerbreadths above the top of patella and therefore check the split through vastus intermedius a trifle higher up (Fig. 74, A).

If we delaminate the tendon of the quadriceps, we can—in case of need— detach the pouch from bone.

A broadly bladed osteotome, close against the shaft and moving

distally, will take advantage of the lucky weft of fat that lies
between the bone and pouch,—a thing to practise first upon
cadavers, for round the uninfected knee we should not make
too bold with cobwebs.[1] Displace the flaccid pouch towards the
joint and so get access to the lower end of shaft.

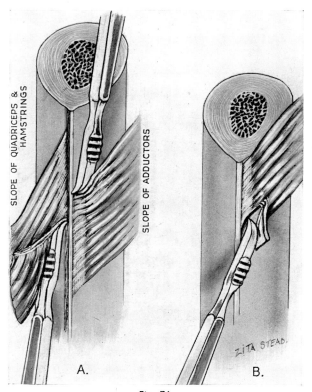

Fig. 76
Stripping the femoral shaft of muscle
A. Work the rugine into the acute or stripping angle which
muscular attachments make with bone, *i.e., up* the shaft for all
the muscles excepting adductors. Note how the rugine tears
into muscle when used in the wrong direction (B) against the
obtuse angle.

Retraction of the halves of intermedius will presently reveal a
foot or more of shaft—a wide span plus a handbreadth (Fig. 75).
But first it must be cleared of muscle.

Stripping the femoral shaft.—The slope of muscle varies : vasti
and the short head of biceps travel down *from* the femur ; adductors, *to* the femur. We strip them off most cleanly by working
the rugine against the *lesser* angle which the fibres make at their

[1] Attempts at separating pouch from *quadriceps* will nearly always tear the pouch.

attachments—the stripping angle of the muscle. Used in the opposite direction the instrument will tend to leave the shaft and tear the fibres—especially at linea aspera where rugged edge and toughly planted tendon contribute (with the effort they evoke) to sharp and sudden deviations (Fig. 76, B).

Beginning at the inner side detach from linea aspera the origin of vastus medialis, which forms the medial intermuscular septum (Poirier) by working *up* the bone ; then separate adductors in the opposite direction.

On the outer side of shaft the rugine works in one way only—

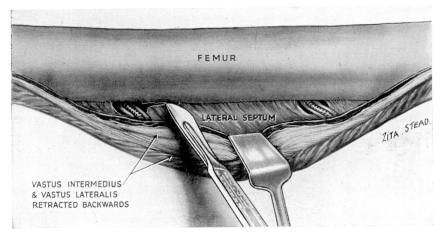

Fig. 77

Stripping the shaft of lateral septum

(The sleeve is open and the femur stripped of quadriceps.)   Sit looking level with the bone. Press back the vastus lateralis and outer moiety of intermedius. Find the perforating bundles coming through the septal archways. The pressure on the muscle draws the vessels back sufficiently to let a *knife* divide the septum from the linea.

upwards : at first against the vasti origins ; and presently—behind the septum—against the shorter head of biceps.

The *lateral intermuscular septum*, irregular in grain and giving passage to the perforating vessels, requires special treatment. Sit looking level with the wound and *see* the vessels coming through their roomy archways. Retraction of the vasti will draw these vessels back sufficiently to let you *cut* the septum close to bone and leave them safe (Fig. 77). (A surgeon, Maurice Pearson, in South Africa—*British Medical Journal*, 1930, **1,** 910—has paid this femoral approach the compliment of making it a ' one-man job '. He has devised retractors (Fig. 78), weighted at the ends, which lever up the shaft and press the muscles back.)

Drainage.—Counter-openings, too, are made with perfect safety by cutting down upon a forceps passed between the outer part of vastus intermedius and the bone. The outer face of lateral septum shuts the forceps off from the sciatic nerve (Fig. 79) and guides it back to skin behind the field of operation. For with the limb recumbent the

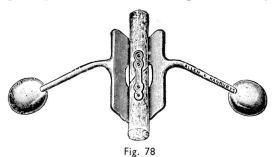

Fig. 78

Maurice Pearson's retractors

These are self-retaining ; they lift the shaft, press back the muscles, and take the place of an assistant.

(The block for this figure has been kindly lent by Messrs Allen & Hanburys.)

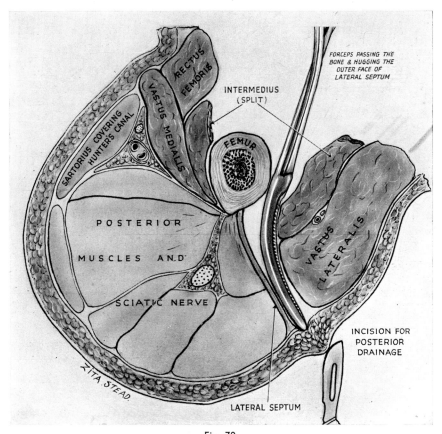

Fig. 79

Posterior drainage after anterior exposure of femoral shaft

When you have ripped the seam and split vastus intermedius slide a forceps past the outer side of shaft, and make it hug the outer face of septum till the skin is bulged behind. Note how the septum buffers the sciatic nerve.

septum is approximately vertical—a statement true of every portion that we use in making *this* exposure. The reason seems to be as follows. Close to the knee for a few fingerbreadths the septum keeps a frontal plane and faces fore and aft; that is because the mass of quadriceps in front of it is almost equal to the biceps mass behind. But farther up the thigh the quadriceps preponderates so quickly as to turn the septum back into a plane that faces right and left. I stress the point to meet suggestions that exposure of the femur from in front is incompatible with proper drainage.

Fig. 80, Part 1

Incision including knee joint with anterior femoral exposure

The black line shows the incision for separate exposure of the joint. The knife avoids the tibial tuberosity.

Extension of Anterior Femoral Exposure to the Knee Joint.—The distal part of this approach is easily continued with the wide benign exposure devised by Timbrell Fisher for the knee joint.[1] He brings his own incision down along the inner edge of the patella. Let us, instead, continue ours along the *outer* edge (keeping, like Fisher, clear of tibial tubercle so that the scar will not be knelt on). This outer cut lies parallel to the main cutaneous nerves and is remote from the medial, transversely placed saphenous branch whose injury gives trouble after meniscectomy. Bring the cut a fingerbreadth below the level of the tubercle (Fig. 80). Reflect the skin medially and expose the *inner* edge of patella; expose also the inner edge of quadriceps tendon to the height of four fingerbreadths. Then split the fibrous covering of the patella along the middle line; reflect the cover inwards just beyond the margin of the bone; cut along that inner edge into the joint. Continue this cut upwards (avoiding inner vastus) through the *tendon* of quadriceps sufficiently to let us dislocate the patella (strung between ligament and tendon) so that its articular face rests on the outer side of outer femoral condyle. Flex the knee to a right angle and make the joint yawn. I have used Fisher's fine, original exposure to pick

[1] *The Lancet*, 1923, **1**, 945.

shot-gun pellets from the back of a condylar recess, and also—
with the trivial change described above—for excising knees through
straight incisions (p. 7).

Repair will (if we wish) seal the cavity with three staggered rows of suture. Drainage can be got in the face-down position— the only way (without resection of a condyle) of using gravity to empty pools in either blind posterior pouch. But drainage damns the knee joint to adhesions; and where the joint and not the life is threatened, as happens often in the early case of knee infection, I have secured quick healing and good function by injecting 10-15 c.cm. of mercurochrome (1 per cent. in water) after thorough aspiration of pus, repeating the procedure three or four times with two-day intervals. Mercurochrome, I found, was harmless to the joint, and was bacteriostatic in that dosage. (This was before the advent of more recent

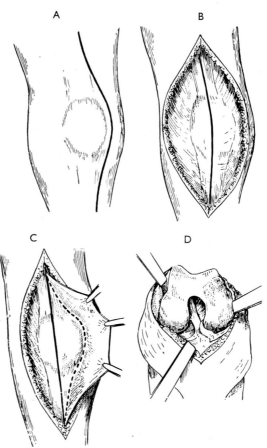

Fig. 80, Part 2

These four drawings, copied by kind permission of Mr A. G. Timbrell Fisher and of *The Lancet*, show that author's original wide exposure of the knee joint through a medial skin incision, A. The procedures figured in B, C and D— reflection inwards of the prepatellar fascia (B), medial arthrotomy (C), and lateral luxation of patella, with flexion of the joint (D)—can all be performed through the *lateral* incision continuing anterior femoral exposure (Fig. 80, Part 1).

drugs about whose action on and in synoviæ I have no personal experience.)

THE UPPER PART OF THE ANTERIOR FEMORAL APPROACH

Let us consider certain details of a region shared by this exposure of the femur and by Smith-Petersen's exposure of the hip.

The fascial webs.—After we part the muscles and move towards the femoral neck, two, three, or four superimposed and separate layers of fascia, remarkable in strength and shape, cross the path of the knife. These layers occupy the space between the origins of the rectus femoris and tensor fasciæ muscles, uniting the *deep* aspects of their sheaths (Fig. 81). Each—like the web between two ' Victory ' fingers—is furnished with a clear-cut margin, concave distally. *One* of the webs (but which, it is impossible to prophesy) has on its deeper face and near its edge an artery the size of radial —the ascending branch of the lateral circumflex ; so it is well before we cut the webs to clamp their margins till we find the vessel.

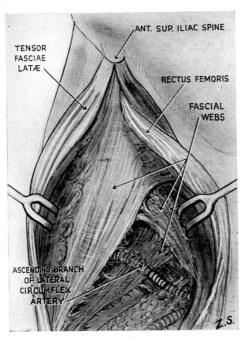

Fig. 81

The fascial webs

These cover the front of hip joint and join the deep aspects of the sheaths of rectus femoris and tensor muscles. Note the relation of web and artery.

The double bonnet.— These web-like structures screen the joint in front. When they are cut a finger-tip pressed firmly on the capsule can just squeeze in above its upper face and force a path between the capsule and a hood which covers it—a double hood or bonnet formed by gluteus medius and minimus, whose deeper part (the minimus) is moulded down in stream-line on the joint. So, to expose the deep articular machinery we raise the bonnet (Fig. 82).

ANTERIOR APPROACH TO THE FEMUR COMBINED WITH SMITH-PETERSEN'S EXPOSURE OF THE HIP JOINT

These two are complementary procedures, a fact of special value in a fracture dislocation (Fig. 82).[1] And so in passing from

[1] Referred to in a paper on that subject (*British Journal of Surgery*, 1934, **22**, 205) written with Bayumi. Mahmud Bayumi died in 1940, only a short while after the Royal College of Surgeons of England had conferred his Fellowship without examination,—a good friend, a loyal follower of Sir Robert Jones, and pioneer in Egypt of common sense in orthopædic methods.

the femur to the hip continue the incision to the level of at least the highest point of the iliac crest—four fingerbreadths behind the anterior superior spine. Then you can raise the twofold gluteal bonnet and turn it back sufficiently to bring the deeply situated hip joint to the *surface*. For that you must, if you are working in the opposite direction (from joint to femur), be sure to rip the seam between the rectus femoris and vastus lateralis at least a wide span

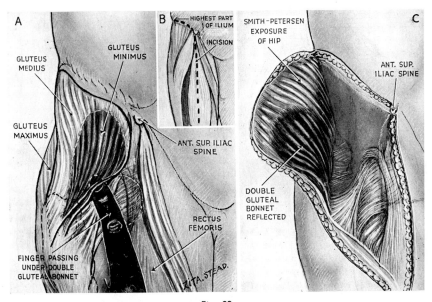

Fig. 82

The double gluteal bonnet and the combined approach to hip and femur

A. Gluteus medius fits over minimus to cover the top of hip joint. B. The incision. Note that it must reach (1) the highest point of iliac crest ; (2) at least a span, distal to the anterior superior spine. This lets you hinge back the muscles sufficiently to bring both joint and femur to the *surface*. C. Shows how the anterior approach to femoral shaft merges with the Smith-Petersen exposure of hip.

distal to the ' spine '. A skimping of the wound, in either case, will leave this deep joint cribbed about by muscle.

I have preferred to *cut* away the glutei from crest and outer face of ilium, instead of peeling off the periosteum : the knife leaves two things that are useful—a carpet on the outer face of ilium ; a fringe along its crest. The fringe will serve for reconstructive suturing ; the carpet lets us catch with ordinary forceps divided vessels in its pile of cut gluteal fibres. But if instead we peel the muscles off, we set ourselves the task of stopping bleeding from a *bone*.

Repair.—Sutures at the crest of ilium bring the great mass of muscle back in place, and pressure keeps it there. Healing is sound in young or old ; for fleshy fibres cut from bone (unlike a tendinous detachment) unite again both fast and well.

EXPOSURES OF THE POPLITEAL FACE OF FEMUR

This face can be approached and dealt with from the inner or the outer side ; or from the back. Each mode of access has its use. That from the *inner* side is not so easily continued up the shaft : the field is crossed by major vessels which must be mobilised and looped away (p. 117).

The *outer* access on the other hand can be at once prolonged far up the thigh—with due respect for perforating vessels. A medial or lateral sinus requiring excision will frequently decide our choice of route.

Fresh injury, again, may need the third or *mesial* approach, but use of it in face of fibrous matting courts danger to the nerves and vessels. Then, too, a hypertrophic scar may form behind the knee—a chance event, outweighed by ease of access and facilities obtained in tracing nerves and vessels up or down the limb ; the place in that respect, is like a no-man's land through which attack may go in two directions. (Description of this midline route comes later—with the calf, p. 135.)

THE INNER (MEDIAL) APPROACH

A plan intending to exploit the rear of any situation solely from the flank might seem a hopeless paradox. But in our surgical assault we hold this clear advantage over generals—the *place* can turn obligingly and let us in.

Try it yourself—or on a skeleton—while one (or other) lies upon the back with limbs extended. Rest the outer edge, say of the *right* foot on the left shin, letting the right knee sag. This turns the popliteal face towards the left—round, nearly, through a right angle. Then, with a sandbag, raise the other buttock (or decorously tilt instead the pelvis of your skeleton) : the popliteal surface turns still farther round and looks not only left but up, towards the ceiling.

The vessels and the bone.—In all exposures of the popliteal face we must negotiate the popliteal *vessels*. That is made easy by a thumbwide gap which parts the vessels from the bone and owes existence to the fact that while, above, the trunks lie close against the shaft, below, the condyles (bridged, of course, by capsule) fend both artery and vein away from femur—much as a backward flexion of the fist will fend a ruler, lying lengthwise, off the dorsum of the carpus (Fig. 83).

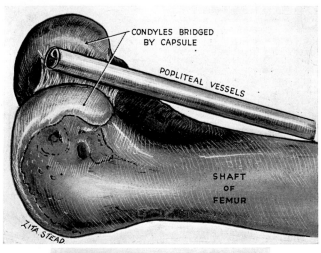

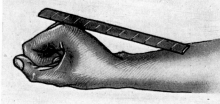

Fig. 83

Showing how the bridge of capsule between the condyles fends the vessels off the popliteal face leaving a useful thumbwide interval.

The *guiding tendon of the adductor magnus* is overlaid by muscle ; sartorius and gracilis cover its medial side. But, when the knee is bent and fascia divided, these bellies slip right back and show the tendon ; only a loose, thin membrane just behind this whitish cord remains to part us from the popliteal space.

THE OPERATION

Position.—A sand-bag underneath the buttock of the sound side tilts the recumbent patient. Place the foot of the affected

limb so that its outer edge rests on the other shin as near the knee
as possible[1] (Fig. 84).

Incision.—Cut *lengthwise* for an ample span, crossing adductor
tubercle. The knife follows the bend of the limb and only severs

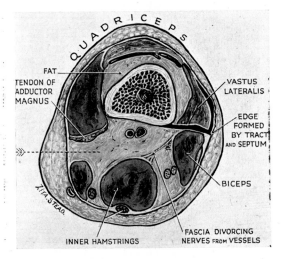
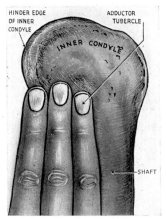
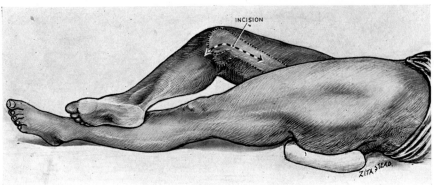

Fig. 84

Position and incision for inner popliteal approach

The knee is shown raised in order to demonstrate the incision clearly ; in practice it rests on
the table. Note above a three-finger method of locating adductor tubercle. When the
' free ' edge of the hinder finger is at the hinder edge of inner condyle the pulp of the anterior
finger covers the tubercle. Note, too, the way in, as shown by the arrow in the cross-section.
(This has been adapted from Eycleshymer and Shoemaker, Section 88, p. 291.)

skin and surface fat. Three fingerbreadths of this incision are
distal to the tubercle, the rest and major part is proximal (Fig. 84).
Be careful here : a medial condyle has often been mistaken for
adductor tubercle ; incisions then lie too far back. Locate the

---

[1] If the knee of the affected side does not flex easily, work from the *opposite* side of the
table.

hindmost margin of the condyle ; the tubercle is found three fingerbreadths in front (Fig. 84).

Dissect the lower edge of skin back for about an inch ; expose sartorius above the level of the adductor tubercle ; divide the fascia in front of it ; then (with Mayo scissors ' on the flat ') detach the deep surface of the muscle, avoiding thus a risk of injuring synovial membrane that lies between the condyle and sartorius.

The free sartorius falls back and leaves exposed the guiding tendon of adductor magnus in front of which the large saphenous nerve leaves the canal of Hunter. The nerve is sometimes carried off upon the deeper aspect of sartorius ; or else lies loosely, strung across the wound. With it is found the superficial branch of the genu suprema artery—the old anastomotic. The *deep* branch of this vessel runs along adductor tendon surrounded by some fibres of the inner vastus. Nor do we see the great saphenous vein (which lies upon the surface of the sartorius), if we have rightly placed our skin incision.

Immediately behind the adductor tendon pick up and open the loose thin fascia—the last impediment before you reach the fossa. Slide a finger in, keeping its back against the tendon, till you touch the centre of the popliteal face (Fig. 85). The *vessels* lie, we know, a thumbwidth from the bone, so bend the finger-tip to find them. Widen the entry to the space and let the finger mobilise the vessels —up to the opening in the adductor magnus, down to the condyles of the femur. As we retract them gently back some twigs they send to bone string out across the wound and thus are easily controlled and cut. The popliteal face of the femur then lies bare (Fig. 85). (The major *nerves* do not appear in this exposure ; they run remote from bone and from the surgeon, p. 123 and footnote to p. 125.)

THE MEDIAL ROUTE EXTENDED TO FEMOROPOPLITEAL TRUNKS AND TO THE SHAFT.—Prolong the upper part of the incision *towards* the mid-point between anterior superior spine and pubic symphysis—in the direction of the femoral artery (Fig. 86). Find the anterolateral edge of the sartorius ; liberate and move the belly inwards off the membrane roofing Hunter's femoral canal. Then split the roof and find the vessels. When the knee is bent the femoropopliteal trunks will come to hand with gentle separation and be loose enough to loop aside. The *outward* twigs which moor the bundle here are few and widely spread ; one set of these, much larger and more constant than the rest, lies about seven fingerbreadths above the adductor tubercle. A little blunt dissection made along the leash and on the outer aspect of the parent bundle will let us raise the major vessels like a bucket-handle and clear an access to the shaft.[1]

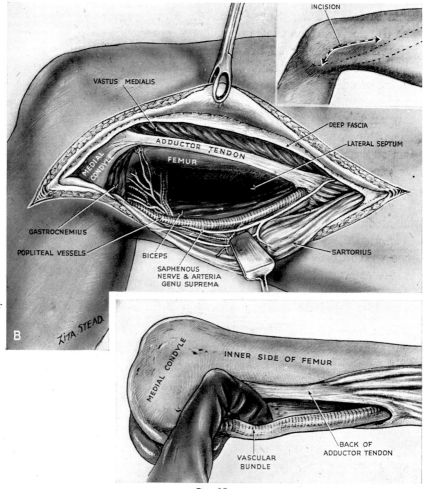

Fig. 85
Exposure of the popliteal face from the inner side

A. Open the flimsy fascia just *behind* adductor magnus tendon ; slide a finger into the fossa keeping its back against the tendon ; touch the *centre* of the popliteal space. Hook the finger to locate the vessels. Widen the opening and mobilise the vessels. B. The popliteal face exposed.

[1] *Mutual relations of femoropopliteal vein and artery.*—Sartorius will help us to remember them : down the *thigh* sartorius and vein have *opposite* relations to the artery. So, where sartorius is lateral, near Poupart's ligament, the vein is medial ; in Hunter's canal sartorius lies in front, the vein behind ; beside the popliteal face of femur sartorius is medial, the vein is lateral. Still farther down, within the bottle-neck produced between the condyles and the heads of gastrocnemius, the vein—as if perforce—lies close behind the artery. But in the *leg* it holds once more a medial position—just as it does near Poupart's ligament.

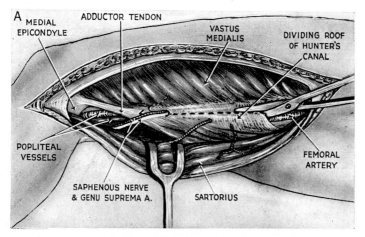

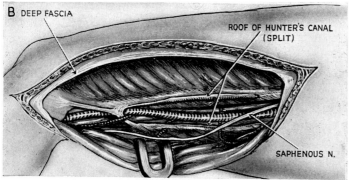

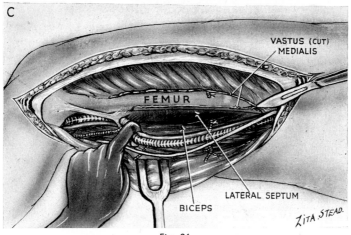

Fig. 86

**Extension of the medial approach to expose first the femoro-
popliteal trunks in continuity, then the shaft**

A. Displace sartorius from the roof of Hunter's canal which is then split.
B. Bend the knee and mobilise the femoropopliteal trunks. In doing this
the leash of very large vessels which binds the trunks to vastus medialis seven
fingerbreadths above adductor tubercle can be cut, or liberated with Mayo
scissors. (In the figure it is cut.) C. Loop the main trunks aside—like a
bucket-handle—and clear a path to femoral shaft.

Then, working at the *back* of the vastus medialis, detach the muscle from its slender hold on bone ; for there, as if to help us, the fibres spring from linea aspera and cover, but have no attachment to, the inner side of femur. So, by a mere extension of the route of Fiolle and Delmas, we expose a span or more of shaft in continuity with popliteal surface.

THE OUTER (LATERAL) APPROACH

Exposure of the popliteal surface from the outer side is simple. We take advantage of a loop-hole leading straight into the fossa, and widen it to reach the bone.

ANATOMY

The loop-hole.—Close to the condyle the shorter head of biceps lies ' free ' behind the septum, and there a touch—once fascia is opened—will separate the belly and reveal (between the biceps, the septum and the condyle) a loop-hole opening in the popliteal fossa —a crevice we shall presently enlarge (Fig. 87). But we must find it first. And what a mess if we should fail ! For cuts that blunder into quadriceps through tract or septum will sometimes cause a singular confusion, incredible till actually seen.

The iliotibial edge.—Mistakes, for once, are almost inexcusable. We can enlist the certain guidance of a hard and constant edge which marks the union (at an angle) of lateral septum with the hinder margin of the iliotibial tract (Fig. 87). The *edge* will therefore lead us in behind the septum to the loop-hole.

We have a choice of ways for finding it. The wise use both.

THE TWO-FINGER METHOD.—With the knee partly flexed run your middle and index fingers (side by side and touching) *lengthways* down the outer surface of the thigh—your left fingers for the left thigh, your right for the right. When the tip of your middle finger touches the back of the fibular head the pulp of index rests on skin that shifts across the stable hinder edge of iliotibial tract (Fig. 87). Behind this edge (which merges, inwards, with the septum) is a loose, soft mass of biceps—so different with anæsthesia from the cord we feel behind a wakeful knee.[1]

---

[1] The biceps ' tendon ' just above the joint is *not* the cord-like structure which often seems so obvious to eye or touch. It is instead a *lamina* that coats a wider belly and goes slack with it. " *Les deux portions de ce muscle s'attachent à l'extrémité supérieure du péroné par un tendon considérable qui monte en s'élargissant derrière ces deux portions réunies.*" Little escaped the Baron Boyer.

THE TEST OF RELATIVE MOBILITY.—Grasping the soft and mobile biceps belly close above the condyle we find it moves across the stable edge (Fig. 87). This simple test will guide our knife and bring us opposite the loop-hole.

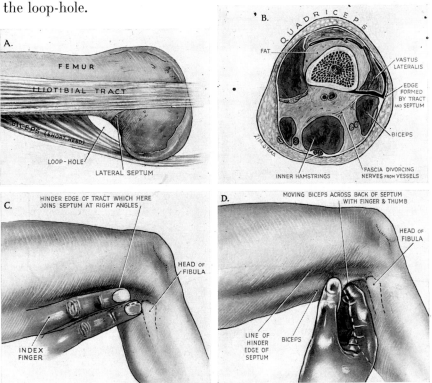

Fig. 87

The outer popliteal approach

A. The loop-hole. B. Cross-section showing how the guiding edge which lies in front of the loop-hole is formed by the junction of iliotibial tract with lateral septum. At this low level (but not higher up) tract and septum form a right angle. C. *Two-finger method of finding the edge.* Use right middle and index fingers for the right side, left for the left. Slide them lengthwise down the thigh till the tip of middle finger strikes the back of fibular head. The pulp of index feels the edge. D. *The test of relative mobility.* Find the edge by moving biceps across the back of septum.

The biceps, passing to the fibula, crosses the outer head of the gastrocnemius, and, on the outer side of lateral condyle, lies for a little space against the synovial membrane of the knee—a fact to keep in mind.

THE OPERATION

Position.—Place the patient on the sound side with the sound limb straight. Lay the knee of the affected side just before its fellow knee so that the heel will rest on the ' sound ' shin and tilt the popliteal face to a convenient angle (Fig. 88).

Incision.—A longitudinal cut a span in length—through skin and fat but *not* through deeper fascia—exactly maps the hinder, guiding edge of the iliotibial tract, down to the head of the fibula (Fig. 88). Make *doubly* certain of this guiding edge before you seek the loop-hole. Then, close above the condyle, pinch up fascia just behind the edge ; divide it lengthwise with the edge as guide. A finger-breadth above the condyle a touch with Mayo scissors will detach the ' free ' part of the biceps belly from the septum and reveal the loop-hole. (Avoid the use of pointed scissors which might prick synovia round the condyle.)

Enlarge the loop-hole with the finger. Work gently up along behind the septum, and free the slight attachment of the biceps. As you do this you meet with two or three resistant strands—twigs which the perforating vessels give to biceps before they pass (through septal arches) to the quadriceps (p. 124). Divide and tie these twigs. Avoid the cramp of working

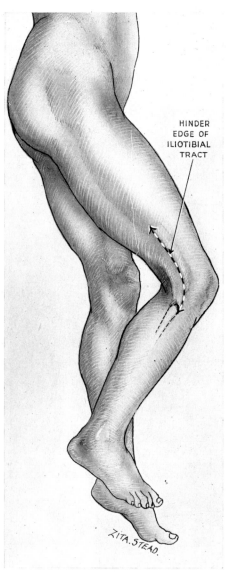

HINDER EDGE OF ILIOTIBIAL TRACT

ZITA. STEAD.

Fig. 88

Lateral popliteal exposure

Position and incision. The *position* serves, too, for exposing fibula (p. 161 below).

down a pit by separating the biceps upwards to the *limit* of your skin incision. Then through the gap slide in a finger close above the condyle, keeping its back against the hinder surface of the septum. Touch with the nail the centre of the bony plane, and hook the finger gently to catch and mobilise the rope-like parcel of the vessels ; divide a few unpaired and variable offsets that moor it loosely to the femur. Retraction then displays the popliteal face in full (Fig. 89).

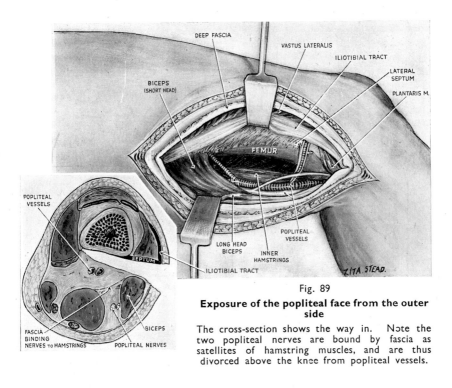

Fig. 89

Exposure of the popliteal face from the outer side

The cross-section shows the way in. Note the two popliteal nerves are bound by fascia as satellites of hamstring muscles, and are thus divorced above the knee from popliteal vessels.

The major nerves—like persons with too many aliases [1]—keep in the background : reaching the fossa from behind, they lie, as one might guess, behind the vessels (which reach it from in front). The nerves, in fact, are satellites of the hamstring bellies and have (above the knee) a mere, and easily divorced, *proximity* to vessels. That is why, when the popliteal artery and vein are hooked up by a finger, the nerves are unperceived and left behind : until they reach the leg, a sheet of intervening fascia postpones the linkage which creates a neurovascular bundle (Fig. 89, inset).

[1] For comment on these aliases see p. 127 and footnote, p. 128

THE LATERAL POPLITEAL ROUTE EXTENDED TO THE OUTER FACE OF SHAFT.—Ten inches more of femur can be seen by this extension. No main trunks cross the field ; we deal instead with transverse branches of the perforating vessels (Fig. 90).

Let us continue the incision of the skin (p. 122) a handbreadth

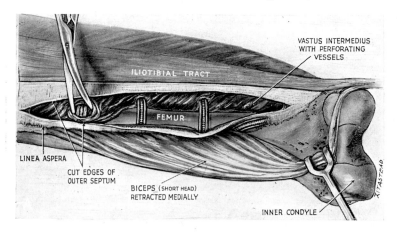

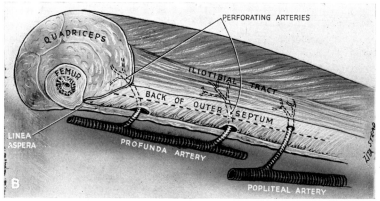

Fig. 90

Lateral popliteal exposure extended to the shaft of femur

A. Split the outer septum lengthwise from behind. Trace the ladder-like lay-out of vessels through the vasti ; then work between the ' rungs ' and bare the bone.
B. Shows the anatomy in diagram.

up beyond the length of shaft we wish to bare ; and, in the same direction, pursue the stripping of the biceps from septum and (as well) from the linea. This will expose the naked back of the septum.

The vascular bundles.—The terminals of perforating vessels from profunda cross the field to reach the outer vastus group in series with some lower twigs that spring from the popliteal trunks. But none—except this lower singleton or pair—are obvious : *it* runs a little way in view before it perforates the back of septum, contrasting thus with branches of the profunda that disappear, as soon as they have crossed the linea, through septal *arches* ranged along the shaft.

If then we split the septum lengthwise from behind, we come directly on the *back* of the quadriceps (on the vastus intermedius below, and half-way up the shaft, on the vastus lateralis, Fig. 71, D). Beginning at the linea we trace the bundles through the rather open texture of the vasti. A very little care will keep the vessels safe while a rugine strips off the flimsy hold of muscle from the outer side of shaft.[1] This leaves the bone conveniently accessible between and underneath the bundles, which now lie spaced like ladder rungs across its naked flank (Fig. 90). And, if we wish, we can divide a rung or two.

REFLECTIONS ON RELATED POSTERIOR EXPOSURES IN THIGH AND LEG AND ON THE LEG IN GENERAL

An old approach of Guthrie's through the calf—a method which of late received new life and grace—gives origin to several exposures. In these we separate the heads of the gastrocnemius, proceeding proximally for the thigh, distally for the leg. Attack on either part where it adjoins the other will of necessity involve the fellow segment; for nerves and vessels hold so fast in each that if we limit our approach to leg or thigh we cannot mobilise the neurovascular ' bundle '.[2]

The ' bundle ' dominates the popliteal space; control of it is

---

[1] The clearance of the *inner* face of femur from the back is troublesome; it is most difficult in the approach to peel off tough insertions of adductors without progressive injury to major veins. For, with the patient prone, the perforating vessels are jammed between adductors and the femur. In contrast it is simple, as we have seen, to push these vessels backwards—clear of bone—when working from the front (p. 108).

[2] '*Bundle.*'—We have already noted (p. 123) as a point of practical importance that popliteal nerves and vessels are divorced above the knee; they therefore fail (above the knee) to constitute a veritable neurovascular bundle. The fact is obvious when we approach these structures from the *side*: the finger hooks up vessels only, for fascia segregates the nerves and binds their trunks as satellites to hamstrings (see the cross-sections, Figs. 87 and 89). That, we saw, is why the nerves elude our search in medial or lateral approach. But if we enter from the back and reach as deep as popliteal vessels, we must in doing so destroy the crucial sheet of thin, divorcing fascia; and then—when that is gone—the mere proximity of nerve and vessels will let us hook them up collectively in what *appears* to be a bundle. (This note explains why ' bundle ' has inverted commas here, and below, pp. 135, 137.)

vital, whether we wish to deal with its constituents or draw it sideways from our path.

The gastrocnemial heads.—First we must separate these heads which are surprisingly disposed ; for though the widest part of femur lies between their origins, they do not form, as that might lead one to expect, a long V pointing down the limb.   Instead they

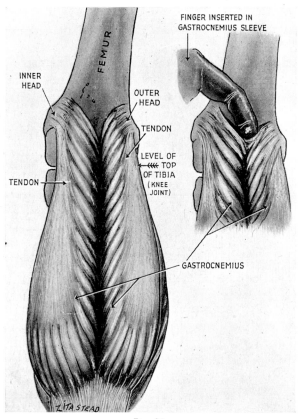

Fig. 91

Showing how the gastrocnemius V is formed *above* the level of the knee joint.   A finger can define the V which marks the entrance to the half-sleeve covering the back of leg.

meet before they leave the thigh and make a shallow midline V above the joint ; and there, if other guides default, a finger may be hooked between the heads (Fig. 91).

The mesial guides.—The early union of the heads gives value to the guides that help in parting them below ; for swollen calves are soon deformed by posture, and midline structures shift.   Two guides—a vein and nerve—will almost always set us right : they mark the groove between the bellies of the gastrocnemius—the seam to rip, Fig. 92. The vein (the blue guide) is the short saphenous ; it rests on fascia covering the groove. (A deep elastic layer of superficial fascia—the kind used recently in plastic work—invests the upper reach of short saphenous vein. Preserving fluids rich in phenol sometimes make this layer simulate deep fascia ; the vein

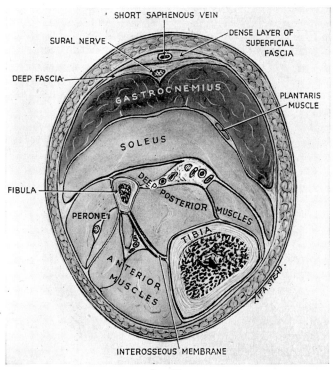

Fig. 92
Guides to the gastrocnemius seam
Note how the blue guide (short saphenous vein) is bridged by deep fibres of *superficial* fascia which bind it to the surface of deep fascia. (Sometimes the vein is deep to deep fascia.) The white guide (sural nerve) is regularly deep to deep fascia and *occupies* the groove between the gastrocnemial heads.

then seems to occupy a level deeper than they say it should—a thing it *really* does quite frequently. My thanks are due to the Dominions officers who put me wise to this.)

Another guide (the white) lies in the groove itself, and thus within the envelope of fascia. It is the sural or calf nerve which like its inner fellow was also called saphenous from association with a vein too often far too obvious. This nerve springs from the tibial, once called internal popliteal : more distally, near tendo

Achillis it gets a strong communicating branch from common peroneal (once called external popliteal).[1]

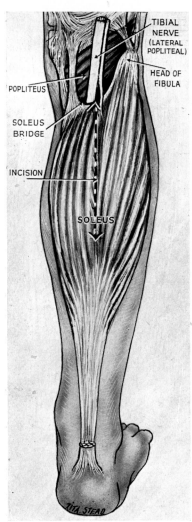

TIBIAL
NERVE
(LATERAL
POPLITEAL)

HEAD OF
FIBULA

POPLITEUS

SOLEUS
BRIDGE

INCISION

SOLEUS

RITA STEAD

Fig. 93
The soleus bridge

The main vessels pass deep to it—between calf muscle and deep muscular group. Note where the large muscular nerve enters the edge of the bridge.

The half-sleeve and the striped seam.—The gastrocnemial heads unite to clothe the calf with a half-sleeve which we can lift with ease from underlying structure. The seam, we know, is doubly striped —in blue and white. Ripping the seam we find the popliteal bundle which goes from view beneath the slanting archway of a bridge formed between tibia and fibula by soleus belly (Fig. 93). The grain of soleus is chiefly longitudinal ; so we can split the bridge and find the bundle deep to it. Nothing could be easier ; the shade of Guthrie (with whom Larrey walked arm in arm through Cairo wards) might well rejoice. His method has survived the interlude when men, perhaps like Hunter's pupil, earned it the title " bloody ", ranking the muscles " beefsteak number one "—and two and three.

The riddle of the bolster leg.—Indeed, this wide approach should have displaced by now the medial and cramped exposure in the calf, so indirect, so cherished by examiners,

[1] Rehearsal of these aliases is due to recent efforts aimed at making us *un*learn. We are to scrap, it seems, the painfully acquired (but excellent) " tibial " and " common peroneal " of the B.N.A. ; so that, once more, internal (or medial) popliteal must change —invisibly—within a single segment of the limb and call itself posterior tibial, merely to suit the very questionable naming of an artery (see p. 130). The tibial plays no such tricks, and " peroneal " marks the striking early difference in course between its own deep branch and vessels *afterwards* related. Calling the other peroneal branch " the superficial," in place of musculocutaneous, prevents (I know) uncertainty regarding site—in arm, or leg—when looking through the journals.

Alice, again, in *this* peculiar nightmare, might compromise with popli-tibial, and popli-fibular.

so blind and therefore dangerous. For who knows what may lurk in swollen limbs from raid or accident ? " A lucky-bag " was Ryall's word for the abdomen;[1] and, in respect of chance variety, the bloated calf becomes a kind of belly. The whole traumatic list of ' closed ' conditions must be long for I have seen the following myself : a fissured fracture causing bleeding from the arch of anterior tibial vessels, which formed a clot that blocked the crural circulation (see p. 151) ; a bruised arterial trunk with distal vasoconstriction ; aneurysm of the peroneal artery due to a broken shaft of fibula that wrenched away a *distant* branch ; the bursting of some forty varices (with no arterial injury) caused by the pressure of a wheel ; a gross œdema of each separate muscle (this in the upper limb) associated with constriction of main arteries to twine-like thinness. (The size and pulse of these diminished vessels were suddenly restored after a major slitting of fascial wrap and sheaths of muscle.)

A medley such as that in bolster limbs may wear a common mask of swelling and defective circulation, but any wholesale swaddling of these injuries in plaster—without the benefit of open exploration—will hold as grim an outlook as it would for sets of dubious ' acute ' abdomens.

Tracing the bundle down the calf, we saw, was simple ; to trace it midway up the back of thigh is simpler still. For hamstrings part behind the knee, and we prolong their separation. We shall exploit this facile cleavage in amputating through the thigh with aid of local block, reducing hæmorrhage as though we used a tourniquet ; which we shall not (p. 138).

A GLIMPSE OF LEG

Leaving the no-man's land behind the knee let us revive a general acquaintance with the leg, not troubling greatly over detail.

The calf we have already seen ; the two great muscles, gastrocnemius and soleus, sandwich plantaris. We saw the neurovascular bundle pass beneath the bridge of soleus; there it assists in marking off the bunched mass of the calf from the flat length of *deep* posterior muscles. Let us observe the vessels first.

The main vascular bundle and its distal fork.—Once more we

---

[1] Sir Charles Ryall (1869-1922), remembered for his work on the danger of implanting cancer cells during operative interference, and better still for the affection in which he was held by his colleagues.

are the dupes of terminology. " There is," we learn, " a main popliteal trunk that ends at the distal edge of popliteus ; there it divides into posterior and anterior tibial arteries." " Posterior tibial," we are told, " goes on a small way down and then gives off the peroneal branch " —a mere collateral one might assume. We get no picture of the facts as seen by surgical approach.

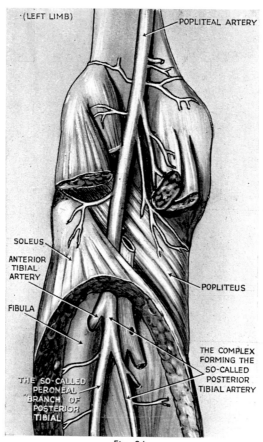

Fig. 94
The popliteal artery as currently depicted
(This is the only *left-limb* figure I have used. The drawing is after the relevant portion of Fig. 761, p. 794, Gray's *Anatomy*, 27th Edition, 1938 ; the indications have been modified.) A picture typical of many books, which rightly contradicts their texts : it shows conditions seen alike by artist and by surgeon—a main stem going down *beyond* its forward branch to end below by forking. (The texts end popliteal artery at anterior tibial and lump the rest of stem plus half the fork as ' posterior tibial,' having as ' branch ' a vessel often larger than itself—the peroneal.) But artists, too, are fallible. The picture we have copied makes, like many others, anterior tibial come from the *side* of popliteal ; in my experience (and Boyer's), it springs from the front—a point of surgical importance (pp. 151 and 152).

Looking afresh with those whose drawings contradict our texts (Fig. 94) we, too, shall see a stem—which is a ' main' —descending through the popliteal fossa, passing the popliteus muscle and going on some finger-breadths to end by forking sharply *like a catapult* —with larger emphasis at times on one or other side. That forked arrangement must be frequent : apart from absence of posterior tibial vessels in a single leg there has been no exception in the last thirty cadavers I have seen. That, too, is what a master of anatomy, the Baron Boyer, saw and described in 1815 (Fig. 95).

" And what," you will ask, " has become of the *anterior* tibial artery ? " Well, it is just a branch from the front of a main

stem—a stem which Boyer calls the popliteal down to its
tibioperoneal fork.[1]

We shall show presently how we can draw the proximal part
of this anterior tibial branch right back into the calf and see exactly
how it juts and curves (pp. 152 and 155).

But we are thinking too arterially ; the *veins* are large and thin-
walled, sometimes varicose, outnumbering the arteries by two to

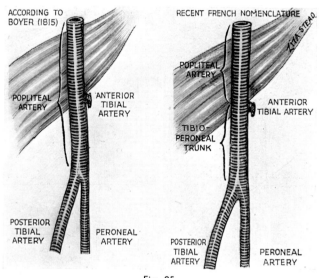

Fig. 95

Nomenclature which fits the distal forking of a main stem.

one. So veins bedevil intervention and complicate our much too
simple picture of a place where vessels fork and arch—in triplicate.

The *distal portion of the bundle*, about the level where gastrocnemius and soleus join with tendo Achillis,[2] edges inwards from
between the deep and superficial muscle layers, and is covered there
by skin and fascia only (Fig. 96). Thence we can trace it up the leg,
detaching as we go the slender mooring of soleus to the tibia, which
may reach down within a handbreadth of the medial malleolus
(p. 147 and p. 148, below).

[1] Since Boyer's day his countrymen, less simply though with clarity, make the popliteal
  end (as we do) at the anterior tibial branch, and then impose the name of tibioperoneal
  trunk on the last fingerbreadths of stem above the fork. We can, with those accounts,
  believe our eyes ; for each describes (as we do not) a major stem that goes *beyond* a
  forward branch and ends below by forking (Fig. 95).

[2] *Tendo Achillis*, changed in B.N.A. to *tendo calcaneus*.—This kind of make-believe at
  growing up is charmingly discouraged in pages cardinal to scientific outlook. " *La
  gentillesse des fables*," wrote Descartes, " *réveille l'esprit* " : their pleasant touch, he found,
  could stir the mind. (*Discours de la Méthode*, Part I.)

Leaving aside for later study the lateral peronei and the popliteus, turn for a moment to the tibial shaft.

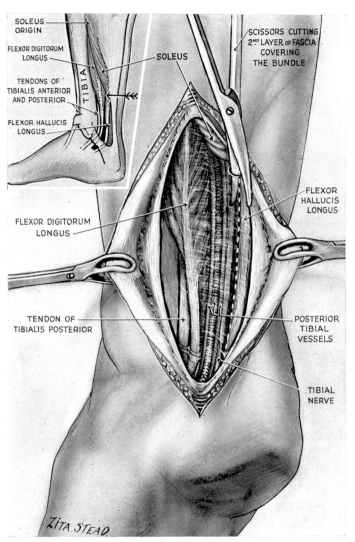

Fig. 96

The distal part of the posterior bundle in the leg

It is covered here by skin and by *two* layers of deep fascia. The inset shows how tibial fibres of soleus cross and interrupt the plane of cleavage between calf and deep muscles—the plane in which the bundle lies. The deeper fascial layer and these soleus fibres serve to moor tendo Achillis more firmly on the *tibial* side : see p. 148. The arrow of the inset points to where the bundle leaves the shelter of the calf.

Anterior and deep posterior leg muscles (Figs. 97, 98).—The subcutaneous surface of the tibial shaft separates a belly of the deep

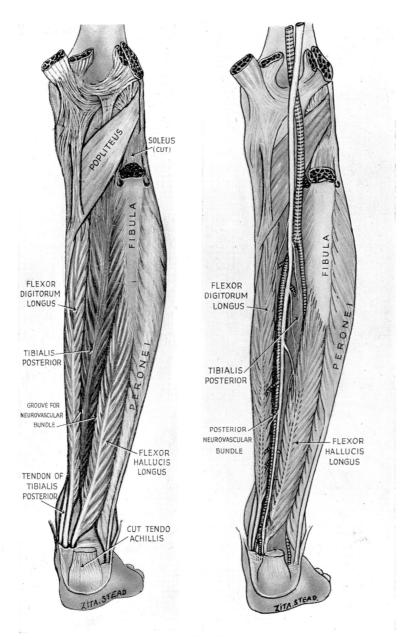

Fig. 97

The deep posterior leg muscles

Note how they form a groove for the posterior neurovascular bundle.

posterior group behind from a belly in front ; of these the anterior
only is called tibialis ; the belly behind is the long flexor of the toes.

The tibialis posterior springs from both bones of the leg ; it is
the deepest belly in the posterior compartment. Its *tendon*, however, comes to the surface by passing inwards deep to the tendon
of the long flexor—a relation of crossed fingers. In the distal third,
therefore, the superficial face of tibia does actually separate two

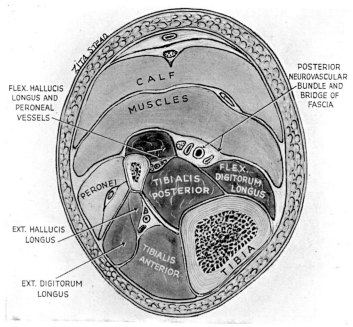

Fig. 98

The relations of deep posterior leg muscles with the anterior group

Note here, too, the groove for the posterior neurovascular bundle. A
bridge of fascia makes the bundle a satellite of the deep group. Note how
the subcutaneous face of tibial shaft separates the *belly* of tibialis anterior
from the *belly* of flexor digitorum longus. (The inset to Fig. 96 shows how
the face of tibial malleolus separates *tendons* of tibialis anterior and posterior.)
Extensor hallucis longus is the only *deep* muscle of the anterior compartment.

structures known as tibial—the tendons, *not* the bellies, of tibialis
anterior and posterior (Fig. 96, inset).

The other muscle of the deep posterior group, flexor hallucis
longus, springs (like extensor hallucis in front) from the middle
two-fourths of the fibula—the ' middle half ', if you reduce the
fraction. The bellies of this flexor and the flexor of the toes
encroach sufficiently upon the hinder face of tibialis posterior to
form a gutter for the neurovascular bundle—a gutter bridged by

thin, translucent fascia which grows thick distally where it escapes the shelter of the calf (Figs. 96 and 98).

Turning now to the *anterior compartment* we find two main superficial muscles, and later we shall look between them for the neurovascular bundle (p. 153). These muscles are (1) the tibialis anterior (whose belly *and* whose tendon flank the subcutaneous face of tibia), and (2) extensor digitorum longus (coming mainly from the fibula). The off-shoot muscle, peroneus tertius—a badge (not always present) which marks us from the apes—springs with extensor longus. The one deep muscle of the anterior compartment, extensor hallucis, arises from the ' middle half ' of fibula. Going obliquely (as it must to reach the inner toe), its belly overlaps the neurovascular bundle and sets a trap (p. 157).

This general and bare account (by furnishing a sort of common back-cloth) will stage in turn exposures of the limb and let us focus on the detail.

THE MIDLINE APPROACH TO THE POPLITEAL FACE OF FEMUR

For this we need add little to the general reflections on p. 125. Here, too, as in exposure from the outer or inner side, we have to mobilise and then displace the intervening ' bundle '. But working this time from the back there is (in contrast with a side approach) no " open sesame " ; the place itself will not revolve and let us in. So we must take it squarely, by direct assault (cf. p. 114).

Incision.—Find first the level of the joint—a fingerbreadth above the head of fibula (Fig. 99). Incise in what you *think* the middle line—a guess which (due to swelling and decubitus) is often wrong. But soon there will be guides. Cut, then, through skin and fat a handbreadth distal to the joint and upwards for a span above its level.

The seam.—Look for the short saphenous vein (the blue guide to the middle line). It lies, remember, deep to fat, along the groove between the heads of gastrocnemius, most often on the surface of deep fascia (but sometimes underneath). If it does not appear at once, reflect a little skin at either edge. The final proof of mesiality, the sural nerve, is constantly subfascial : it occupies the groove (Fig. 100). Open deep fascia behind the calf to look for it, and not behind the knee joint, for there a greater trunk (internal popliteal nerve, or tibial of B.N.A.) lies close beneath investing fascia, and

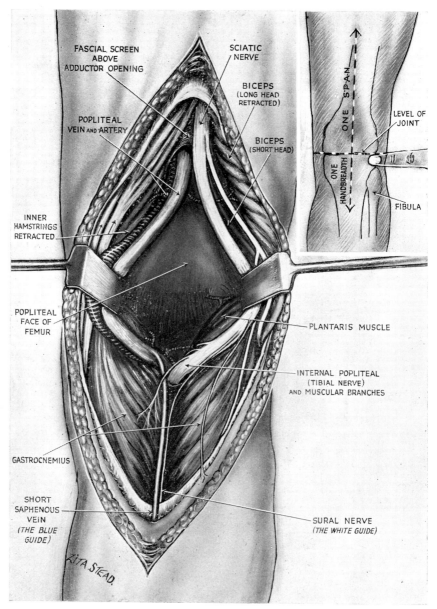

Fig. 99

**Midline popliteal approach.   (The figure gives a cramped and strained impression.
It has been used designedly to show that freedom of the bundle and consequent exposure of the bone will only be secured when we have ripped the gastrocnemius
seam.)**

The long incision lets us mobilise the nerve and vessels : we either draw them bodily
aside or part them (as above), moving the vessels towards the point of their fixation in
adductor opening.

may be ripped in face of extra tension—like cortex under dura. When we have split the seam in gastrocnemius this popliteal trunk becomes a guide to separate the inner from the outer hamstrings ; a finger helped a little with the knife dissolves their slight cohesion.

The ' bundle '.—Retraction of these sundered bellies in the calf and thigh reveals, beneath the inner popliteal (tibial) nerve, the

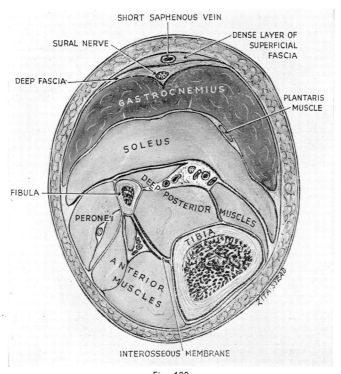

Fig. 100
Guides to the gastrocnemius seam
Note how the blue guide (short saphenous vein) is bridged by deep fibres of *superficial* fascia which bind it to the surface of deep fascia. (Sometimes the vein is deep to deep fascia.) The white guide (sural nerve) is regularly deep to deep fascia and *occupies* the groove between the gastrocnemial heads.

close-knit popliteal vein and artery—the last impediment before we reach the bone. Then—if the finger finds it easy to displace—the ' bundle ' goes *en masse* to either side ; but, if it loosens grudgingly, we humour its constituents and pass between, moving the nerve towards its outer (peroneal) fellow, the vessels inwards—to the side where they are fixed in the adductor opening. The popliteal plane at once becomes accessible (Fig. 99, noting the *legend*).

Bending the knee will loosen everything behind the joint and

let the bone approach the surface. But relaxation sets peculiar
traps, and semitendinosus may drift limply to the middle of the
wound and there be claimed as great sciatic.[1]

EXTENSION OF THE MIDLINE ROUTE.—The distal part of this exposure lets us move the nerve and vessels far enough aside to cut
through popliteus and expose the hinder, ' popliteal ' face of tibia
without dividing the soleus bridge (cf. p. 144 and footnote).

The next few pages show that we can use the mesial approach
(combined with simple lateral posture) in the most frequent
amputation of the thigh—that through the distal half.

A POSTURE FOR THIGH AMPUTATION WITH NO TOURNIQUET USING PROCAINE [2]

Custom has reconciled us to the supine posture for those who
need this amputation. With that disposal limbs are slung from
raised supports ; or else a nurse must bear their weight. In
either case we work at levels awkward for injecting nerves if
spinal block is inadvisable.[3] These troubles vanish when we place
the patient on his healthy side ; then, if the damaged limb will
flex, the nurse need never lift the foot, but only grasp the leg and
keep the heel—as *pivot*—on the table (Fig. 101). She thus presents
each aspect of the patient's thigh : the sides in turn are brought
to face the surgeon ; while to expose the back she lets the knee fall
gently down across its fellow (Fig. 102). So, after infiltrating areas
of flap or cuff, and *all* the operative field—most thoroughly—with
procaine ($\frac{1}{2}$ per cent.), we can in comfort see and block the great
sciatic trunk. While that is growing numb we shall ligate main
vessels and thus avoid the use of tourniquets.

---

[1] I saw this seemingly absurd mistake made twice, by reasonable men—a sign perhaps of
    decent equilibrium ; for those who let us know they are infallible in any field are either
    lunatics, " economists of truth ", or in the even larger class one thinks of as ' unfortunate ',
    which lacks both virtue and the chance to fall.

[2] *The Lancet*, 1940, **1**, 736.

[3] Procaine nerve-block, used alone or in company with gas-oxygen or minimal amounts
    of ether, was strikingly employed by Lotfy Abdelsamie, F.R.C.S., in my surgical unit
    at Kasr el Aini Hospital, Cairo, during work that much reduced mortality from crush.
    Abdelsamie's valuable paper should have new currency in times like this of calculated
    trauma. (*The Lancet*, 1936, **1**, 187.)

The supplementary incision.—For this twin purpose make a *mesial* cut—first outlined by a weal—through popliteal skin one handbreadth distal to the joint and going upward to a spot three fingerbreadths above the site proposed for bone division (Fig. 103). We find the mesial guides (p. 126) and separate the boundaries of the popliteal space ; then we can trace the tibial or inner popliteal nerve up to sciatic trunk, which we inject with

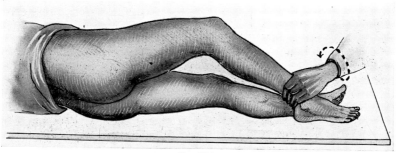

Fig. 101

The flexed limb pivots on the heel, which rests on the table. The nurse holds the leg and rotates it to present the front and sides of the patient's thigh to the surgeon without lifting the limb.

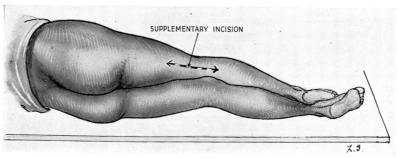

Fig. 102

The knee falling across its sound fellow gives access to the back of thigh. A long midline incision exposes the sciatic nerve for high injection and the main vessels for ligature.

15 c.cm. of a 2 per cent. solution of procaine—first in the sheath, then in the total thickness of the trunk.

Ligation from behind of femoral vein and artery.—The blocking of the nerve affords an interval in which to tie the two main vessels. These run, of course, at deeper levels—near the bone. And though the artery and vein do not officially become the popliteal till they have passed the opening in adductor magnus, yet, as they near the opening, only a trifling web of tissue screens them from the posterior compartment. So, if we trace the vessels *from below* (where

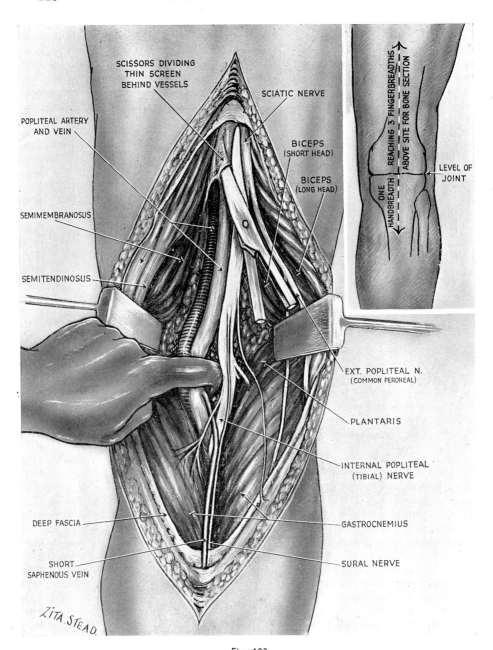

Fig. 103

The long midline incision and its use

A finger introduced at the medial edge of the tibial (internal popliteal) nerve *behind the knee* hooks the main vessels up from the femur. Trace them proximally and tie them *above* adductor opening after dividing the thin fascia which screens them from behind.

we can hook them blindly off the femur),[1] it is extremely simple to disrupt the web and tie them well above the level for dividing bone (Fig. 103). We then proceed according to our training or experience : incisions, joining with the mesial cut behind, run distally and forwards ; the flaps are made and muscles severed.

During these activities, however, the great sciatic trunk will rest in peace—until the time comes to remove the limb. With procaine infiltration not less than twenty minutes must elapse between injecting and dividing this capacious conduit of shock impulse. And that, indeed, is little time enough. Let us recall and profit by two clear and striking facts : our own distress when dentists shorten by a jot the dozen minutes *they* allow for nerves far smaller than the huge sciatic ; the sudden fading of the patients pulse when stimuli get through a partial procaine block, un-supplemented by another anæsthetic.

The method used in the attempt to burke the later growth of axones will have prescribed already the length of nerve we first injected. I do not dare to say which method is the best, for no one knows ; but each will place the procaine to suit his own belief. It is at least important, once the limb is off, not to pull out the severed nerve and cut it short at levels unprotected by the procaine ; though I have seen this done.

We have to deal as well with the *saphenous nerve*. The guide to it—a whitish raphe on the medial side of thigh, found on displacing the sartorius—denotes the tendon of adductor magnus ; a nick with Mayo scissors made immediately in front of this will open the canal which holds the nerve. Then trace it up the thigh, inject it level with sciatic, and divide it when the same long interval has lapsed.

I can confirm Abdelsamie's finding : " Amputation under *full* novocaine analgesia is a benign measure that does not shock the patient."

STUMP SEPSIS AFTER AMPUTATION FOR DISTAL INFECTION

I have seen many thigh amputations performed for this reason with careful technique after scrupulous preparation, but I have also seen, and had myself, too many septic results—perhaps because bacteria from distal foci were travelling up lymphatics during the operation, out of range of chemicals applied only to skin. In my

---

[1] A stress on " from below " is justified : the *fevered* searches that one sees begin high up, where vein and artery are hard to find.

experience sepsis came whether rubber drains were left a long or short time : if long left they seemed to determine infection ; but dangerous pooling of exudate ensued upon early removal. This pooling is prevented by placing ribbon gauze, heavily coated with dilute bipp, as a slender pack under each layer at the time of suture—for example, between bone and fascia (or muscle), and between fascia and skin. The bipped ends of the ribbons protrude as drains, and the pack is so well lubricated that it can be removed painlessly after forty-eight hours. A dry wound is left which will at once be covered with a *thickly* bipped dressing. These drains do not carry in sepsis from without, as rubber may ; and certainly, too, the bipp can check bacterial growth.[1]

A relevant example of its use in another field interested some of my co-workers in this country. The large cavity left by removing a mandibular osteoclastoma was packed with bipped ribbon after thorough treatment of the wall with the high-frequency current. The cavity (lined now with dead tissue) communicated not only with the surface of the neck but also with the mouth, and the patient ate and drank as usual from the day following operation. When we removed the pack for the first time at the end of a fortnight we found a lining of clean red granulations. The pack—except on its oral surface, where saliva had washed out some of the bipp,—was unaltered and fresh like the cavity.

I have no experience of the original bipp, which might be toxic in this quantity, having never used any but the dilute variety, whose value I learnt from Stoney during the last war ; nor have I met with any other preparation which could so triumph in the test just described.

[1] The ingredients of dilute bipp are :—

Bismuth carbonate	.	.	1 part		Hard paraffin	.	.	.	.	2 parts
Iodoform powder .	.	.	2 parts		Soft paraffin	.	.	.	.	12 parts

Its preparation requires careful attention to details, of which R. Atkinson Stoney, of Dublin, has sent me the following note :—

Put the iodoform and bismuth in a large mortar and mix well. Melt the hard and soft paraffin together on a water bath ; stir well and cool slowly, stirring all the time. Take a little of the mixture of hard and soft paraffin and rub it up with the mixture of iodoform and bismuth till a smooth paste forms. Add the rest of the paraffin little by little to make a uniform ointment. The bipp should have the consistence of firm butter and should *not* be greasy. In very hot weather increase the quantity of hard paraffin and reduce the soft. (In wards the bipp is best kept in separate containers for individual patients.)

With this, I must confess, one does not quite recapture the lipstick qualities conferred on dilute bipp by pharmacists in France. But I have left the note—like that of p. 11 concerning compound fracture. For recent drugs are not the first, by many years, to start a habit of obtaining excellent results from wounds, however grossly soiled—which still, I see, claim victims.

EXPOSURE OF VESSELS AND NERVE IN THE BACK OF CALF

Incision.—Find first the level of the knee joint, a fingerbreadth above the top of fibula. A *mesial* incision measured from this

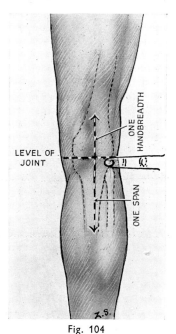

Fig. 104
Incision for midline calf exposure
Note the level of knee joint viewed from behind : it lies one fingerbreadth above fibula.

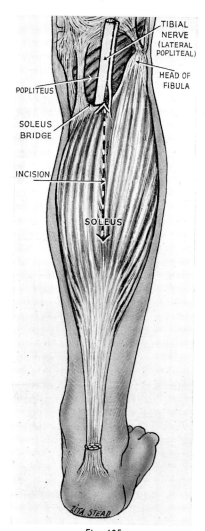

Fig. 105
The soleus bridge
The main vessels pass deep to it— between calf muscle and deep muscular group. Note where the large muscular nerve enters the edge of the bridge.

plane, runs for a handbreadth up the thigh, a span along the calf (Fig. 104). The rest we know : the half-sleeve of the gastrocnemius, striped on its seam in blue and white, and surgically ripped to show the soleus bridge ; the lengthwise splitting of the bridge ; the underlying venous and arterial ' catapult ' (pp. 125-131).

The bridge-mouth of soleus.
—The tibial nerve which runs behind this catapult of vessels bisects their tibioperoneal fork, but first supplies the bridge-mouth

of soleus with a sturdy twig—most easily divided (Fig. 105). And so—before you split the bridge,—define this entrance gently with a finger beside the disappearing vessels. (See that the foot is plantar flexed, and bend the knee to make the wound both lax and shallow.)

EXPOSURE OF THE 'POPLITEAL' FACE OF TIBIA.—This follows the exposure of the nerve and vessels whose bundles we can now displace to reach our first objective—the fan-shaped popliteus.[1]

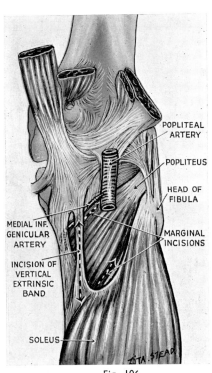

A useful vertical extrinsic band.—The sheath that cloaks the popliteus is strengthened at its widest, medial, part by constant fibres which belong to semi-membranosus (Fig. 106); these cross and stick upon the fan-like grain—a grain that yields when split a glimpse of concave bone through thick and grudging muscle. So for a better view, transect the popliteus. The knife should reach the tibia by cutting lengthwise down the band. A liberating cut is also made, respectively, along the upper and the lower margin of the popliteus. Both liberating cuts should finish *medial* to the middle line; they thus avoid the nerve to popliteus, which lies behind the muscle and ends by curving round its lower border. The upper cut should also miss the vessels (inferior medial genicular) which slope along the upper edge and are attached to it by the extrinsic band of fibres (Boyer). So, with its nerve intact, we mobilise the popliteus, raising it from bone towards the *fibula*. Then there is room to deal with our objective.

Fig. 106

The vertical extrinsic band

The knife transects the grain of popliteus by cutting lengthwise down the band. Liberating cuts are made along the margins of the muscle, sparing genicular vessels above. Retraction of the muscle towards fibula will expose the concave face of tibia. Repair by suturing *across* the band whose fibres stop the creep of sutures.

Labels on figure: POPLITEAL ARTERY; POPLITEUS; HEAD OF FIBULA; MEDIAL INF. GENICULAR ARTERY; MARGINAL INCISIONS; INCISION OF VERTICAL EXTRINSIC BAND; SOLEUS

---

[1] The distal portion of the midline popliteal route (p. 138), which lets us mobilise the barrier of nerve and vessels, will also let us reach this hinder part of tibia—*without* dividing the soleus.

We make a sound repair by suturing the popliteus at right angles to the length of the extrinsic fibres ; for since they cross the fan they stop the sutures creeping through its grain.

EXPOSURE OF THE POSTERIOR NEUROVASCULAR BUNDLE IN THE LOWER PART OF THE CALF AND BELOW

Lesion of nerve and vessels half-way down the leg (or farther) is dealt with through a medial and *long* incision. The distal mark

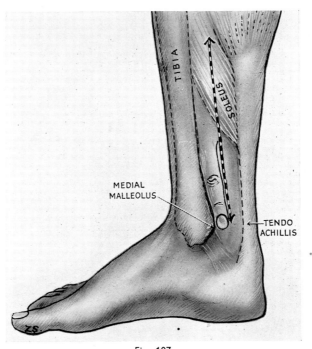

Fig. 107

Incision for the posterior neurovascular bundle of leg (distal half)

The finger with one edge pressed against the back of tibial malleolus marks with its other edge the distal end of the *artery*. Above, the knife avoids saphenous nerve and vein by cutting two fingerbreadths behind tibia. Note how fibres of soleus spring from tibia and cross the plane of cleavage between calf muscles and the deep group.

for this should overlie the bundle. But where—exactly—is the mark ? Many books to-day agree in placing it " midway between the medial malleolus and the tendo calcaneus : "—a reasonable site, unfortunately countered on a previous page of one respected work, which makes the posterior tibial artery end " midway between the tip of the medial malleolus and the most prominent part of the heel." This ancient piece of imprecision (by contrast with its clear-cut fellow) haunts, I find, the memory of surgeons,

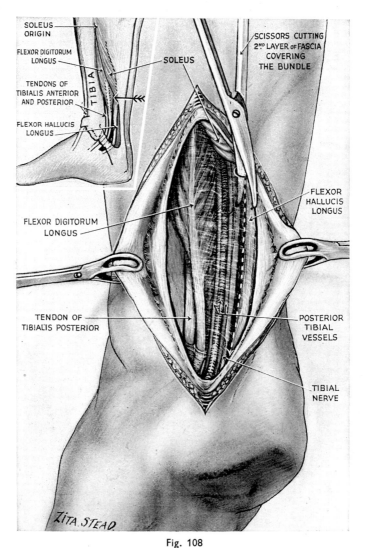

Fig. 108

The distal part of the posterior tibial bundle

Note the thick *second* layer of deep fascia covering the bundle. Above, it thins out to part deep muscles from calf. Divide it *beside* the bundle. To follow the bundle *up*, detach the tibial origin of soleus (inset). The arrow points to where the bundle leaves the shelter of the calf. If you must also reach the level of the ' catapult ' use—in supplement—the midline access (p. 143). (For plantar continuation see p. 163).

and echoes widely in alternatives : " the medial tubercle of the calcaneus " ; " the centre of the convexity of the heel ",—uncertain places, deep to thickened skin, that serve to misdirect incisions and guide them too far back.

Let us forget this careless talk. The vessels lie a fingerbreadth behind the medial malleolus. Try on yourself. Press one edge of a finger down along the *back* of malleolus ; the other edge controls the tibial pulse. The finger therefore marks the *end* of an incision whose purpose is to amplify a plane of cleavage and thus is long enough to show the vessels without exactly following their course (Fig. 107).

Incision.—This will divide skin only. Measure a span extending from a fingerbreadth behind the medial malleolus to reach a point above, two fingerbreadths posterior to tibia—avoiding thus the long saphenous vein and the companion nerve which lies just deep to it (Hovelacque). Open the surface sleeve of fascia and then a *deeper* sheet which binds the bundle to the deeper group of muscles. This second fascial layer while it lies beside Achilles tendon is strong, opaque and tense, but passing under shelter of the calf it there becomes a thin translucent pellicle. Begin dividing it above, for down below the vessels may be slit as they approach the line of skin incision (Fig. 108). To trace it farther upwards use the plane of Fiolle and Delmas in front of the Achilles tendon—a solid strap that lets us lift the calf away from deeper muscles which hold the bundle in a satellite relation (p. 134).

Nothing is perfect : the facile cleavage plane (which, in itself, might symbolise an influence of France on surgical technique) is crossed above by fibres of soleus. Detach soleus from the tibia if you should wish to follow up the nerve and vessels. But soon, as you come up towards the level of the ' catapult ', it will be easier to reach them by splitting through the midline of the calf (p. 143). So, if you must, you will combine these two exposures.

To get the widest field you plantar flex the foot and bend the knee. (Note that the distal portion of the tibial nerve has kept its relative position in the bundle : it still lies just behind and lateral to tibial vessels—exactly as it does when it bisects the catapult.)

Exposure of this hinder bundle is easily continued to the sole, if we should need to trace the plantar distribution of nerve and vessels (p. 163, and *legend* to Fig. 125, below).

EXPOSING THE BACK OF THE DISTAL END OF TIBIA

Mention of the tibia suggests the thought of an exposure from the inner side. But, if we try a simple test, we find we shall do better to employ a *fibular* approach. Kneel for a moment with the foot relaxed in plantar flexion. Then grasp and move the flaccid tendon of Achilles ; it travels farther to the inner side—away from fibula—and so uncovers more of an objective which spreads across the middle line. One reason is that while its outer edge is ' free ', soleus fibres reaching down the shaft (it may be almost to a handbreadth from the medial malleolus) tie the Achilles tendon to the tibia. So, like a dog, it moves most easily towards its leash. Another—dominating—factor is that on the medial side Achilles tendon is more firmly fixed, than on the lateral, against the *denser* portion of the sheet of fascia covering the deeper muscles of the leg (p. 135 and *legend* to Fig. 96, p. 132).

Displacement of Achillis is not the sole advantage of an outer access, for that will let us liberate as well the belly of the flexor hallucis—a muscle which arises from the fibula and spreads at once to hide the tibial surface. This belly (with the aid of a strategic interval) is readily displaced towards the *in*accessible and medial fixation of its tendon down the foot.

Position and incision.—A sand-bag laid beneath the instep of the ' face-down ' patient bends his knee and keeps the foot in plantar flexion. The skin incision curves from a point a full thumbwidth below the fibular malleolus and goes a largish hand-breadth up the leg, close to the outer edge of the Achilles tendon— a line that will avoid the sural nerve which otherwise is likely to be cut above and also distally (Fig. 109, A).

After incising fascia the knife once more will enter fat, crossed as a rule two fingerbreadths above os calcis by an artery, which must be severed ; its parent stem, the peroneal, accompanied by veins that may be very large, lies here on bone and stripes the shaft of fibula just medial to the hinder edge.

A further opening of the fat will show a spot where we can reach the back of tibia, between hallucis and the fibula—an angular strategic interval (Fig. 110, A, inset).

But first be sure you *have* identified hallucis. The common, disconcerting slip is to mistake for it the peroneus brevis whose belly has a way of bulging in towards the tibia. To test the matter embrace the doubtful muscle from behind with thumb and finger ; and if in front of it you pinch the narrow fibula, your grasp includes

not hallucis but *both* the peronei.   The hallucis lies farther in
and deeper (Fig. 109, c).

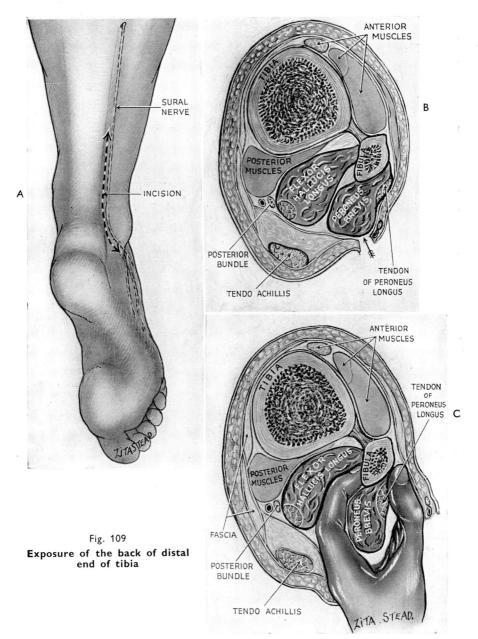

Fig. 109

**Exposure of the back of distal
end of tibia**

A. The incision close and *lateral* to Achillis, avoiding sural nerve.   B. The frequently
deceptive bulging of peroneus brevis that simulates hallucis.   C. Recognition of peroneus
by closing on the narrow fibula in front with an embracing thumb and finger.

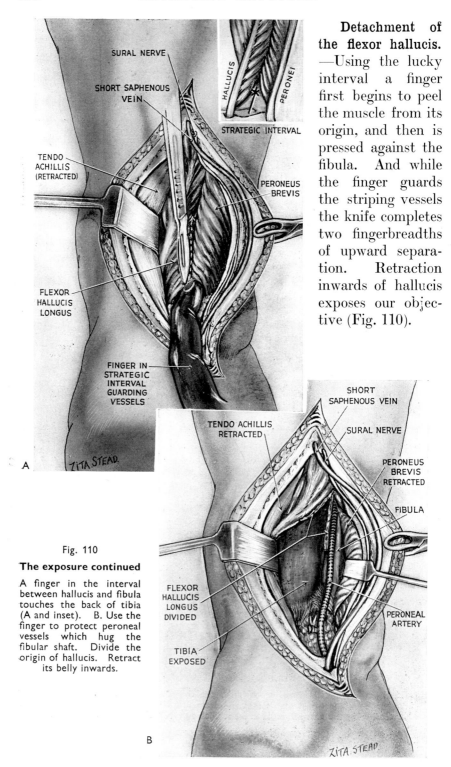

Detachment of the flexor hallucis. —Using the lucky interval a finger first begins to peel the muscle from its origin, and then is pressed against the fibula. And while the finger guards the striping vessels the knife completes two fingerbreadths of upward separation. Retraction inwards of hallucis exposes our objective (Fig. 110).

Fig. 110

The exposure continued

A finger in the interval between hallucis and fibula touches the back of tibia (A and inset). B. Use the finger to protect peroneal vessels which hug the fibular shaft. Divide the origin of hallucis. Retract its belly inwards.

EXPOSURE OF THE ARCHED SEGMENT AND UPPER THIRD ANTERIOR TIBIAL VESSELS [1]

Our study of the *leg* began behind—the master site and starting place of crural trunks ; the answer, thus, to Dupuytren's perplexity when faced with local bleeding : " But *which is cut* ? Is it anterior or posterior tibial ? The peroneal or the popliteal ? One or else several at once ? "

Transition from the back comes easily ; the arching forward of anterior tibial vessels leads straight into the front compartment. Distal to the knee this deep, sequestered segment juts from the popliteal stem, and passing through the interosseous membrane turns down—like a tap.

Records of bleeding from the arch are rare enough to leave at least some surgeons unprepared to stop it by direct exposure. Yet this hæmorrhage is dangerous : the mass of blood (or clot) is placed exactly where it shuts both tap and main as well.

Fiolle and Delmas (1921, *Surgical Exposure of the Deep Seated Blood Vessels*, London, p. 21) describe how Pierre Duval (to reach an aneurysm of the arch) cut through and drew aside the upper third of fibula. For that he bared the bone, dividing peroneus longus, the outer head of gastrocnemius, and part of soleus—liberating first the common peroneal nerve and looping it aside.

The poor condition of my only patient with bleeding from the arching segment led me to try a quick alternative. I therefore used a tiny ' Mikulicz '—a tampon placed exactly where a finger-tip controlled the unseen vessel. But that might sometimes fail to stop the hæmorrhage, or might (like clot itself) impede the circulation.

Looking for other means I found a simple one.

THE OPERATION

With Dupuytren, no doubt, we wondered what was bleeding and have (I trust) begun to reconnoitre from the back. So— through a mesial incision of at least a span—we shall by now have ripped the sleeve of gastrocnemius and traced the popliteal vessels downwards to the bridge-mouth of soleus ; and, if the mouth has overhung and masked the branching of the major trunks, we have already cleared a prospect by splitting lengthwise through the bridge.

But still there is no sight of our objective : the arch juts

[1] *The Lancet*, 1943, **1,** 141.

forward and away. Nor can we yet persuade it backwards into
view, for it is fastened out of reach—in front. And turning to the
front we *there* release the arch and draw it out behind.

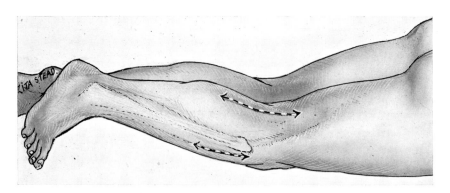

Fig. 111

Exposure of arched anterior tibial segment

With the patient face-down cant the foot across the sound ankle. You then have
easy *simultaneous* access to front and back compartments of the leg.

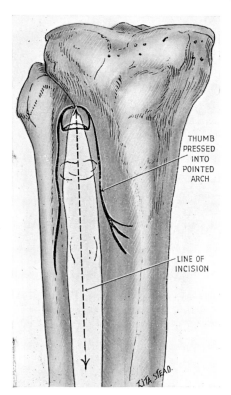

THUMB
PRESSED
INTO
POINTED
ARCH

LINE OF
INCISION

Position.—Till now a sand-bag lifts the instep of the ' face-
down ' patient, bending his
knee to slack the calf. Now
(without altering the posture
of his trunk) take the foot
from the bag and lay its
medial edge across his other
ankle (Fig. 111). The trivial
change gives access to the
front compartment and leaves
the hinder wound in sight
and in control.

Fig. 112

**Finding the intermuscular plane for
opening the upper reach of the anterior
compartment**

The thumb, pressed up from below, fits
lengthwise into the pointed arch between
tibia and fibula. Open skin and fascia
along a line bisecting the thumb from
nail to wrist. The line marks where the
curved plane of cleavage comes to the
surface (see text); it does *not* mark the
course of the anterior tibial bundle which
here lies deep to the lateral muscle.

A rule of thumb for the anterior incision.—First we must separate the pair of muscles that cover the front of the vascular arch and its continuation down the leg. Between the two the

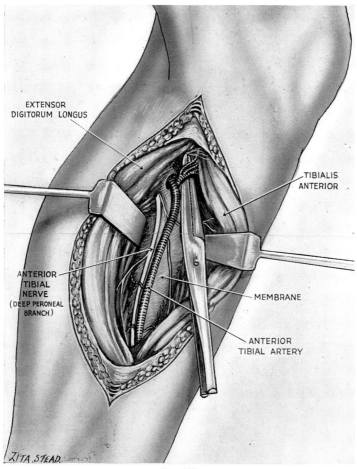

Fig. 113

Cutting the leash of anterior recurrent tibial vessels to free the arch

A pair of forceps slides up the interosseous membrane medial to the main neurovascular bundle and lifts the leash for section. A few small nerve twigs may run with it and can be spared: they do not moor the arch. If they are cut, tibialis anterior remains well supplied.

cleavage plane is *curved* : the belly of extensor longus digitorum bulges into that of tibialis. This curving plane comes to the fascial surface along a line which can be found with ease. Approaching from below press and fit the pulp of your thumb into the pointed, gothic archway formed above by tibia and fibula (Fig. 112). Divide the patient's skin as if you were bisecting the guiding

thumb from nail to wrist—a method of location more robust than
ghostly pointers to the plane of cleavage (the academic groove or
petty artery or whitish line) which soon fade out with trauma.
Using this guide again, we open fascia along the same line, *not*
tearing muscle. A finger separates the interlock of bellies and
shows the bundle of anterior tibial vessels. These are deep to long

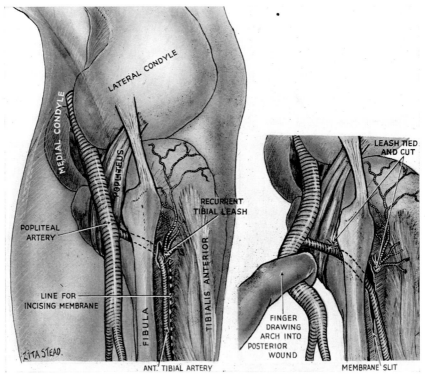

Fig. 114

A. The arch set free in front, and B, drawn back and brought to view in the posterior
wound. A narrow opening through interosseous membrane has been widened medial
to the vessels.

extensor and so lie lateral to our incision (see the *legend* to Fig. 112).
When we have made them visible throughout the wound against
the background of interosseous membrane we can proceed to
mobilise their arch.

Impediments of leash, membrane and muscle.—The arch is
moored in front by its recurrent branch and venous tributaries—
a wide-flung leash whose narrow end we cut (Fig. 113).[1]

---

[1] John Bell—brother to Charles, the physiologist—says of the anterior recurrent tibial :
" It is a branch which comes off the fore part of the tibial artery instantly after it has
pierced the interosseous membrane ; it turns immediately upwards under the flesh of
the tibialis anticus ; it gives many muscular branches, some to the head of the tibialis,

Then, if the opening in the membrane is large enough already, we are at liberty to draw the arch back into the calf. But, if the hole itself is small—or narrowed by encroachment of the hinder tibialis—we must enlarge the passage, slitting the membrane downwards medial to the bundle (to avoid the nerve); and then, if need be, stretching with a finger a pathway through or over tibialis. That will remove the last impediment and let us bring the arch from front to back for safe and unrestricted access (Fig. 114).

EXPOSURE OF THE DISTAL TWO-THIRDS OF THE ANTERIOR TIBIAL NEUROVASCULAR BUNDLE

The long incision of Fiolle and Delmas so greatly simplifies the operation that those who read of it incline to over-confidence. Its virtue dwells in length : it reaches down to where the *tendons* have replaced a close-packed interlock of bellies ; and using tendons we can cleanly split extensor digitorum from the tibialis. So all we have to do is choose correctly. And that is just where many fail : they take a near-by tendon for the tibialis and lose their way at once.

A little care avoids discomfiture. We know (p. 135) that in the leg tibialis anterior borders its namesake shaft throughout : *that* is its certain countersign. The tendon lateral to tibialis (except immediately above the ankle—where hallucis comes forward to replace it) must, during anæsthetic relaxation, be a tendon of extensor digitorum longus ; the interval between is the required interval.[1] But first let us divide the skin.

Incision.—Press—in the distal half of the leg—your *little* finger

others to the upper part of the extensor digitorum, and branches go round the head of the fibula to the origin of the long peronæus muscle. One branch goes directly upwards and spreads all over the front of the knee-joint mixing its branches in the common muscular net-work." (John and Charles Bell, 1816, *Anatomy and Physiology of the Human Body*, London, vol. ii, p. 28.)

[1] The text-books here are rather careless ; or do they merely illustrate once more the striking difference in outlook of surgeon and anatomist ? Their pictures show the tendon of extensor hallucis already flush with tendons of digitorum and tibialis, as high as midway up the leg. But, coming from the *depth* of the anterior compartment and springing from the ' middle half ' of fibula, hallucis (when relaxed) *can* only reach the level of its superficial fellows a very little way above the ankle. The tendons, too, of longus digitorum are often drawn as though they formed a single strap within the leg—another point that might seem trivial were it not misleading. In fact, their segmentation as a rule goes about half-way up towards the knee ; and, even where it fails to be complete, the *signs* of it (as Boyer wrote) are visible—" almost throughout the tendon's length." It would be only fair to mention that Baron Boyer practised as a surgeon and had the chance to guess what surgeons want (Fig. 115).

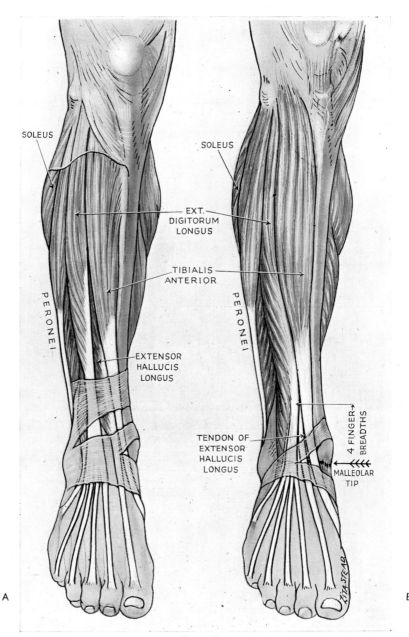

SOLEUS

SOLEUS

EXT.
DIGITORUM
LONGUS

TIBIALIS
ANTERIOR

PERONEI

PERONEI

EXTENSOR
HALLUCIS
LONGUS

4 FINGER
BREADTHS

TENDON OF
EXTENSOR
HALLUCIS
LONGUS

MALLEOLAR
TIP

A

B

Fig. 115

The surfacing of extensor hallucis longus

A is the almost universal picture which affects to show an undisturbed relation, thus inducing surgeons to believe that hallucis reaches the surface midway up the leg and *there* begins to part tibialis anterior from extensor digitorum longus. Anatomists, perhaps, may cock a toe and say (like Galileo) : "But it does !"— unmindful that our patients, properly anæsthetised, do not cock toes. B. Hallucis, when relaxed, comes to the surface three fingerbreadths above the ankle joint. When fully active, tightness of the fascial sleeve combined with structural cohesion will merely let hallucis raise a ridge that carries up a covering of laxer muscles but does not sunder them.

against the outer (fibular) side of tibial crest (or shin). Then ' rule ' a cut along the outer edge of where your finger lay—*not* opening through deep fascia. Cut for about a span (Fig. 116).

The bone and the tendon.—Now for the small precaution. Reflect a little skin at just one distal spot—enough to give a quite indubitable glimpse of tibia. Open the fascial sleeve in line with the incision. The tendon that is flattened close against the bone (and looking rather like it) is tibialis tendon ; the interval we want lies at the tendon's outer edge, and *there* begins our separation.

The last pitfall.—But we can still contrive to go astray. Extensor hallucis, the only deep anterior muscle of the leg, slopes from the fibula to screen the neurovascular bundle. So, if we wander *lateral* to hallucis, we find, perhaps, another artery—or none at all.

You will avoid this terminal collapse by keeping touch with tibialis : work on its outer face, and find the bundle backed above by interosseous membrane, and distally by tibia (Fig. 117). The nerve (deep branch of peroneal, or old anterior tibial), which starts upon the neck of fibula, curves gently in to lie in front of the companion vessels, and then, below, recedes a little out again towards the fibula.

That, at least, is what we learn. Nor can I give at first hand

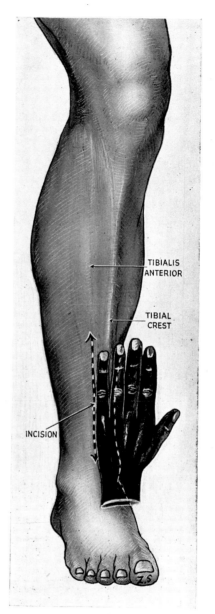

Fig. 116

Incision for anterior tibial bundle (distal two-thirds)

' Rule ' this a little-fingerbreadth to the fibular side of tibial crest. As it goes up the leg, incline the cut towards the bisected-thumb mark of Fig. 112, above. Below, a small medial reflection of skin finds the tibial crest ; next to it is tibialis tendon.

figures to dispute it ; but Hovelacque in his *Anatomie des Nerfs,*
Paris, 1927, p. 609, describes the normal path of the anterior tibial

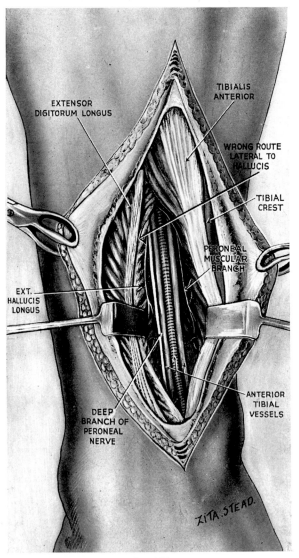

Fig. 117

Showing how the deeply placed extensor hallucis longus
overlaps the bundle. The arrow shows the *wrong* route that
may be taken—lateral to hallucis. (In this figure the nerve lies
lateral to vessels.)

as crossing to the *inner* side of its companion vessels, and shows
this transit at the middle of the leg (Plate LXXXIX). He also
cites Marcellin-Duval who notes that in 450 legs the nerve had

crossed the vessels in all but one per cent. For Boyer, too (in 1815), this transit was the common disposition.

One might from these divergences suspect a strange, cross-channel difference in gross anatomy ; or even that (as Pascal said of truth) *meridians* decide the course of nerves—a thing I rather doubt.[1]

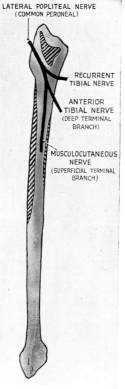

LATERAL POPLITEAL NERVE (COMMON PERONEAL)

RECURRENT TIBIAL NERVE

ANTERIOR TIBIAL NERVE (DEEP TERMINAL BRANCH)

MUSCULOCUTANEOUS NERVE (SUPERFICIAL TERMINAL BRANCH)

Here there is obvious and grave omission. Circumstance prevents me from merging the distal part of this approach into the late Willis Campbell's ' all-purpose ' straight dorsal incision—good alike for ankle and subtaloid surgery. I have used it half a dozen times and seen it used about as often, but too long since to venture, without further opportunity, upon its wealth of detail.

EXPOSURE OF THE FIBULA AND NERVES RELATED TO IT [2]

ANATOMY

The neck and upper third of the fibula are in direct contact with nerves. Muscles surround three-fourths of the shaft.

The relations of the nerves to the upper part of the bone are insufficiently described in many text-books, which give the impression that only the *neck* of the fibula is in contact with the branches of the external popliteal nerve (common peroneal B.N.A.). A glance at Fig. 118 modified from that which accompanies Poirier's excellent account of the peroneus longus,

Fig. 118

Diagram of right fibula (modified from Poirier) showing extent of bone in direct contact with nerves. The shaded areas are the three fibular origins of the peroneus longus. (No other muscle is represented.)

shows in diagram the true extent of this contact (*Anatomie Humaine*, 2ème Edn., vol. ii, fasc. 1, p. 251, Paris, 1901).

It is, of course, at the fibular neck (where the nerves are thinly

[1] The more so since the artist in a recent ' Gray ' refutes the text and shows the nerve as lying *tibial* to the artery within the lower segment of a leg. (Gray's *Anatomy*, 27th Edn., 1938. Compare Fig. 655, p. 649, with the statement in the first two lines on p. 1127.)

[2] Except for the addition of a final paragraph (and the correction of a slip) the text of those pages on the fibula is copied from *Exposures of Long Bones and other Surgical Methods*, Wright and Sons, Bristol, 1927.

covered by the origin of the long peroneus) that they are most often exposed to violence ; but the surgeon whose intervention is not to come within this category should be familiar with the true anatomy of the region.

The external popliteal (common peroneal, B.N.A.) gives off its last three branches as it lies upon the fibular neck : first, the recurrent tibial nerve, which is often double ; then, anteriorly, its deep (or anterior tibial) branch ; and, posteriorly, its superficial (or musculocutaneous) branch. This last nerve descends almost vertically along the shaft, separating the diaphyseal origin of the long peroneus into anterior and posterior moieties, and keeping contact with the upper third of the shaft. Distal to this the peroneus brevis separates the nerve from the bone.

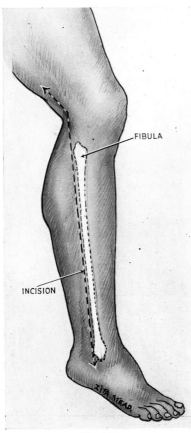

Fig. 119

Divide skin and superficial fascia from the back of external malleolus to the back of fibular head. Continue the incision one handbreadth along the biceps tendon.

Exposure of the upper half of the fibula requires a full mobilisation of these nerves. This can be safely done by defining the trunk of the common peroneal as it descends behind the head of the bone (Fig. 120). When the nerve is raised, it leaves a shallow groove which separates the muscles of the calf from the fibular head. This groove is a strategic point, and gives the surgeon entry to a plane of cleavage which allows him to separate the peronei from the soleus muscle, and thus expose the bone with least damage. In exposing the distal half of the fibula a plane of cleavage between the peroneus brevis and the extensor muscles can easily be found at the apex of the triangular subcutaneous area, but an exposure along this line should be limited to the distal half of the bone.

The following is a description of a complete exposure of the fibula.

THE OPERATION

Position.—The patient lies on the sound side with the sound limb extended. Place the knee of the affected side just in front of the other knee so that the heel of the affected side rests upon the other shin (as in Fig. 88, above).

Incision.—(Fig. 119). Divide the skin and superficial fascia from the back of the external malleolus to the back of the fibular head; continue the incision along the biceps tendon for one handbreadth beyond this. Open the deep fascia proximally, at the medial edge of the biceps tendon; continue its division with blunt-nosed scissors down behind the fibular head. Find the common peroneal (lateral popliteal) nerve where it lies flush with the tendon at the inner side of the biceps insertion. The tendon overlaps the nerve in the proximal part of the wound (Fig. 120). Mobilise the nerve proximally till a loose loop of it can be drawn out across the tendon and the fibular head. Slip one blade of the scissors down

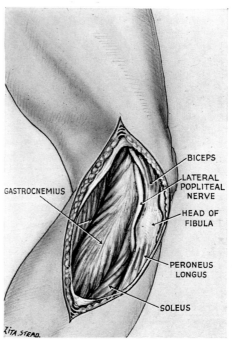

Fig. 120

Open deep fascia over the biceps tendon. Expose the distal end of the outer popliteal nerve (common peroneal); it lies in a groove which separates soleus from the fibular head. **This groove is the key to the plane of cleavage between the peronei and calf muscles.**

along the groove which the nerve has left. Divide the deep fascia in the direction of the groove, and thus open the plane of cleavage between the soleus and the peroneal muscles.

Next, draw the nerve-loop distally (towards the foot); turn the knife's edge away from the nerve against the lower border of the fibular head, and divide the thin slip of peroneus longus which bridges the nerve as it branches upon the fibular neck (Fig. 121). The nerve-loop can thus be drawn still farther out and away from the bone, while the peronei are raised after it and turned forward.

II

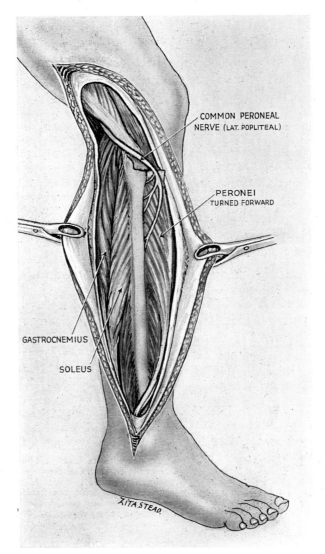

Fig. 121

Mobilise the nerve and lift it from the groove behind the head
of fibula. Slip one blade of blunt-nosed scissors into the groove
and divide the deep fascia throughout the wound. Separate
soleus from peroneus longus. Draw the nerve-loop distally.
Turn the knife edge away from the nerve, and cut through the
thin slip of peroneus which bridges it. Detach the peronei and
turn them forward, keeping the nerve-loop taut.

Stripping the rest of the shaft.—When we have safely bared the upper third of fibula the major task is done, but we should finish well and leave no scarecrow, distal spectacle of ragged bone and tattered vessels. Two sets of things demand and rarely get attention : the different stripping angle for muscles and interosseous membrane ; the close adhesion of the peroneal vessels to periosteum —a contact that begins about a handbreadth distal to the knee.

The *muscle fibres* from the fibula stream towards the foot ; the edge of the rugine should therefore travel kneewards, into their narrow angle with the shaft. At the fibular malleolus, pass the rugine deep to the tendons of peroneus longus and brevis *from behind*. Used from in front and working up the limb the handle of the instrument might strain emerging branches of the musculocutaneous (much better called the superficial branch of peroneal), just where the nerve is liable to form neuralgic trigger-spots.[1]

The *peroneal artery and veins* are seen to hug the lateral malleolus just medial to its hinder edge. A lengthwise cut through periosteum lets the rugine displace them safely from the shaft in company with flexor hallucis. Clean the whole shaft of muscle, working towards the knee. Till that is done do nothing to the *interosseous membrane* ; its fibres slope in the reverse direction ; so you can strip the membrane *down*, towards the foot.

EXPOSURE OF PLANTAR STRUCTURES

Except for pointing abscess, incisions through the sole are best avoided ; they give no comprehensive view, and cicatrise at times with deeply creviced, cornifying scars. Convenient and benign approach is made from the inner side of the foot, or is continued there from the leg (p. 147, above, and *legend* to Fig. 125, below).

---

[1] *Mononeuralgia in the superficial peroneal nerve.*—In 1941 I saw three patients thus afflicted whose *only* pains were in that distribution. These were made worse by turning in the foot with plantar flexion—an act which stretched the nerve ; and, during lulls, pains could be sharply reproduced by pressing on it near but distal to its exit from deep fascia. The nerve just there is clothed in fat, and this—in all three patients—was full of hard and tiny nodules, each very sensitive to needle-prick.

These patients all attributed their pains to sudden twists of foot or ankle. Two were sufficiently improved by procaine ; the third for whom injectional relief had shrunk from weeks to hours, was cured by nerve resection at the trigger-spot.

II*

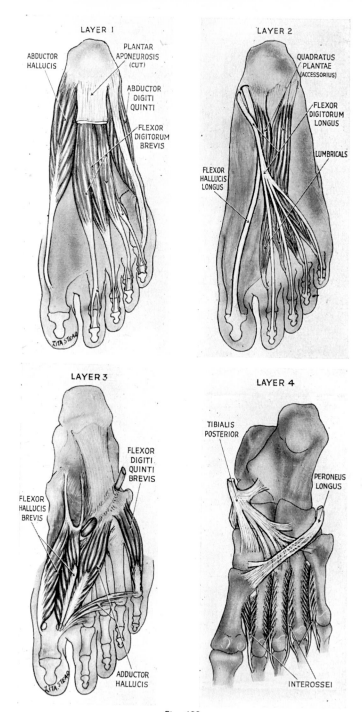

Fig. 122

The four plantar layers

The odd numbers, 1 and 3, are symmetrical with central and flanking
bellies; the even numbers, 2 and 4, have each two long tendons and
short muscles. Layers 3 and 4 lie to the *front*—except for slips from
tibialis posterior.

ANATOMY

The muscles.—Seldom do we find so many grouped as if to aid the memory; and here, yet once again, *muscles* (and their tendons) are the key to surgical exposure. They lie in layers— 1, 2, 3, 4, counting from skin to bone. Layers 1 and 3 (the odd numbers) are both symmetrical: each consists of three muscles —a central belly flanked by two companions. Layers 2 and 4 (the even numbers) differ from 1 and 3 but are themselves akin : each consists of two long tendons plus short muscles (Fig. 122). The layers alternate as follows :—

Layer 1 (symmetrical

ABDUCTOR OF GREAT TOE	FLEXOR DIGITORUM BREVIS	ABDUCTOR OF LITTLE TOE

Layer 2 (Two long tendons   +   Short muscles)
    Flexor hallucis longus   *Lumbricals*
    Flexor digitorum longus   *Quadratus plantae*
                                (=*accessorius*)

Layer 3 (symmetrical)

SHORT FLEXOR OF GREAT TOE	ADDUCTOR HALLUCIS	SHORT FLEXOR OF LITTLE TOE

Layer 4 (Two long tendons   +   Short muscles)
    Peroneus longus   *Interossei*
    Tibialis posterior

It must be noted that (with one exception) the various components of layers 3 and 4 are placed towards the *front*, and are related thus to metatarsal bones and to the distal row of tarsus. So, in the hinder portion of the foot, (where 3 and 4 are absent) constituents of layer 2 must lie next ligament and bone, with here and there an intervening slip of tendon from tibialis posterior (Fig. 122)—the one exception just referred to.

The door of a cage.—The foot when standing on a level surface forms with its skeleton a vaulted cage that opens widely at the inner side. The door which keeps it closed is the abductor hallucis of layer 1 (Fig. 123); and if we free the upper fastenings of abductor and hinge the belly solewards, then we can reach the contents of the cage; though, for the moment, these may be screened by fascia; and even when we open it the muscles are so packed and linked that, till we part them cleanly, the view is worthless.

The long tendons of layer 2 and hallucis brevis.—These are
the bonds which hold the plantar layers close against the tarsal
vault and bind them to each other. The master knot controlling
this assemblage is found about a thumbwidth lateral to the navicular tubercle. Here, where the tendons cross (with hallucis above
the digitorum), they both are tied against the summit of the vault.
Here, too, and just outside the crossing of the tendons, the origin
of flexor hallucis brevis (Fig. 124) suspends its fellow structures ;
for this intrinsically trifling belly procures through its relations a

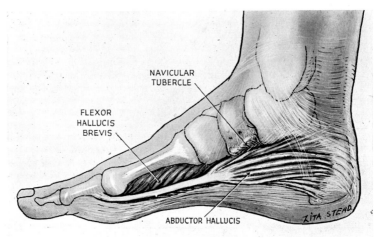

Fig. 123

The cage door

The cage is opened by hinging abductor hallucis down through a right angle
on a plantar hinge. Note the relation of abductor with flexor brevis. Deep to
abductor is a sheet, more aponeurotic than fascial, which sometimes comes
away with the belly but often stays behind and partly screens the cage.

veritable nexus of the first three layers—the three which chiefly
count in this approach.

It happens thus. The tendon of flexor hallucis longus lies in a
lengthwise groove on brevis' belly and straps it to the plantar face
of first metatarsal. Next to, and sometimes joining with, the
inner side of brevis is abductor hallucis of layer 1—an intimate
relationship which often leads to tearing of the brevis belly during
the opening of the cage. Then, on the outer side, adductor hallucis
is sometimes linked with flexor brevis—a chance event that turns
to our advantage and lets us move both muscles solewards as a
sheet which bears off on its plantar face (besides the tendon of
hallucis longus) the lumbricals arising from the fan of longus
digitorum tendons.

If therefore, working on the master knot, we first set free the two long tendons of the second layer, and then the origin of flexor hallucis brevis, we can at once retract a major bulk of muscle from the tarsus and leave the plantar ligaments exposed.

THE OPERATION

Position.—The foot lies on its outer edge ; the knee is partly flexed.

Incision.—Divide the skin and superficial fascia at the inner side of the foot, from the ball of the great toe to the heel, by an incision curving up to cross the tuberosity of navicular (Fig. 125). Identify and catch the veins.

The guide to the cage door.—Find the tendon of abductor hallucis at the inner side of first metatarsal. Mobilise the tendon, taking care to leave intact adjoining fleshy fibres of flexor hallucis brevis. Use the tendon as a guide for separation of the less distinctive margins of abductor belly. Detach this belly, first from its fascial bond with the navicular tuberosity, then from the indefinite anterior part of

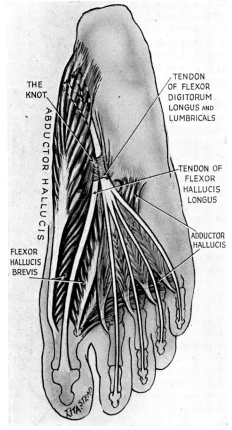

Fig. 124

Flexor hallucis brevis

A vital link of layers 1, 2 and 3. Note the relations of the belly. Its tarsal *origin*—by means of tails, or by a fusion with the fibrous screen *deep* to abductor hallucis—shares in the master knot that fastens long hallucis and digitorum tendons to tarsus.

the vague annular 'ligament' (laciniate of B.N.A.).[1] Continue the detachment down to the inner tuberosity of calcaneus. *Then* you can hinge the muscle solewards through a full right

[1] " Its proximal border . . . is very imperfectly defined. Its distal margin but little more distinct, being continuous more or less with the tendinous origin of the abductor hallucis which arises from it." (T. H. Bryce in Quain's *Elements of Anatomy*, 1923, 11th edn., p. 248.) This band is now appropriately termed *flexor retinaculum*.

angle (Fig. 126), taking care to save the pair of twigs it gets from the medial plantar nerve. Both twigs lie fortunately close to the hinge, two and three fingerbreadths respectively behind the tuberosity of navicular.

The screen, the ‘knot’ and the neurovascular bundles.—When that is done we see the partial screen of fascia, rough perhaps with broken fibres of abductor. The fascia is defective fore and aft, and aft of it we can locate the plantar nerves and vessels. These form two bundles, medial and lateral. Find where they first

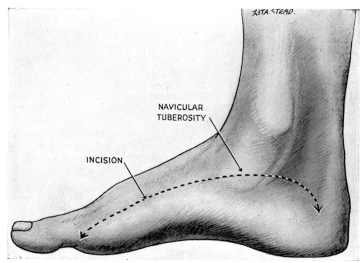

Fig. 125

Divide skin and superficial fascia from the ball of the great toe to the heel. The highest part of the incision crosses the scaphoid tuberosity. Reflect the skin flap downwards and find the tendon of abductor hallucis at the inner side of first metatarsal.

Should there be need to trace nerves or vessels from leg to sole, turn the incision *up the leg*, instead of down the heel. This will leave ample room for skin reflection—sufficient even to ‘decorticate’ calcaneus.

diverge, three fingerbreadths behind the tuberosity of navicular; then they are covered by the screen, and this we must divide.

Next we cut loose the master knot, a thumbwidth lateral to the tuberosity of navicular, dividing first the fibres which attach the two long second-layer tendons to the vault, and after that (a trifle farther out and forward) the strap-like origin of flexor hallucis brevis. Then we can draw the muscles solewards and trace the nerves and vessels on the dorsal side of layer 1.

The *medial bundle* skirts the inner aspect of the long hallucis tendon, and after that runs forward in a gutter thinly roofed by fascia. This gutter lies upon the *dorsal* face of layer 1—between abductor hallucis and flexor digitorum brevis. The *lateral bundle*,

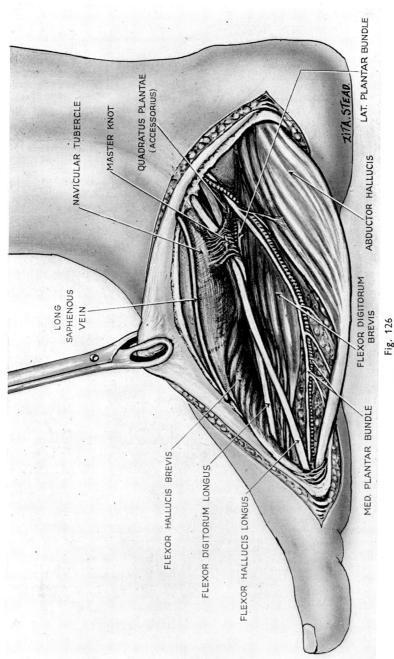

Fig. 126

Plantar exposure

Abductor hallucis has been hinged down through a right angle ; with it has come the fibrous screen. When that occurs you see *at once* the crossing of the two long tendons (flexor hallucis and digitorum), a thumbwidth lateral to navicular tubercle. Take care not to injure the medial plantar bundle near the hinge. The parting of the bundles lies three fingerbreadths behind the tubercle.

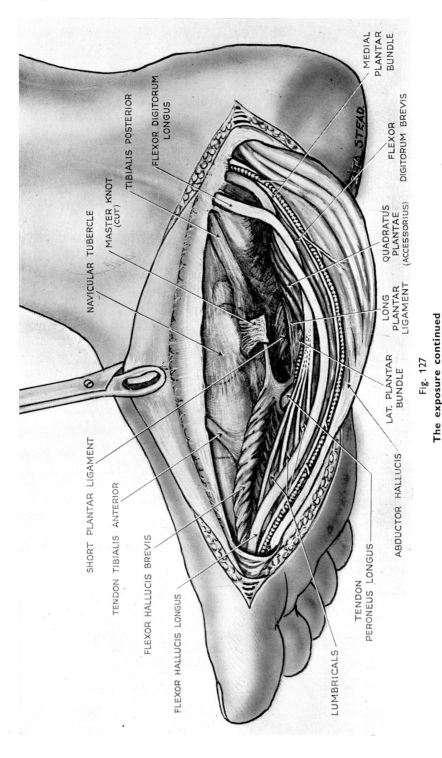

Fig. 127

The exposure continued

The master knot consisting of fibrous derivatives (from screen or from flexor hallucis brevis) has been detached from tarsus letting us retract layers 1, 2 and 3 sufficiently to show ligaments. Most obvious of these is the short plantar. Only the hinder end of hallucis brevis has been disturbed.

slanting out towards the base of fifth metatarsal, skirts the inner surface of quadratus, then lies within a fellow gutter bounded here by flexor digitorum brevis and abductor digti quinti. Reaching the outer metacarpal base, part of the bundle curves once more, but this time inwards. A portion of the outer bundle, therefore, passes *twice* across the sole : first out, between layers 1 and 2 ; then in, between layers 3 and 4. The fact, perhaps, of chief importance is that both the plantar bundles (in the especial segment of their course which can be mobilised most easily) are linked *as satellites* with layer 1. So, when we part this layer from the tarsal vault the bundles too will move away.

Ligaments.—The first to come in view is the *short plantar* ; its fibres slant towards the great toe between the *long plantar ligament* laterally and the ' *spring* ' *ligament* medially (Fig. 127). This last (the inferior calcaneonavicular), by fusing at its inner edge along the base or distal margin of the deltoid ligament, forms a resilient hanging shelf suspended from the medial malleolus. The strap-like tendon of tibialis posterior loops round beneath the shelf, and thus combines to bear the weighted head of talus.

The structures of the sole are now at our disposal and further steps will vary with the object of procedure. Whatever that may be take care to leave the field as dry as though it were the site of toxic goitre : the sponge of venules which infests the foot tends, if it can, to seep in aftermath. And so where circumstance allows, and if you have the right to treat the individual and not the mass, drain, when you close the wound, as you would drain deceitful dryness in a thyroid bed, and raise the fixed and firmly bandaged foot. Then, in a day or two, when drains are out—but not till then, unless you tolerate or disregard *occasional* calamity—then only will you seal the limb in plaster.

It is the fate of detailed ' practical ' descriptions to wear the desultory look of curves mapped out with points : each is a series of related but disjoined minutiæ—the " static snapshots " which the mind demands before it can proceed to the direction of a complex, uninstinctive act. So, it is both a consolation and a stimulus to be aware that in the due performance of the act itself (as in the swift, unhurried hands of surgeons like de Martel) " there is no detail." And closing thus these pages have acquired merit ; they chance to link the memory of two great gentlemen—de Martel's and Roy Dobbin's.

INDEX

Date Due

21			